living well with social anxiety

Praise for Living Well with Social Anxiety

"Do you get anxious in social situations, or care about someone who does? This invaluable book helps you understand this common difficulty and lays out concrete steps you can take to overcome it. People can break free of anxiety by making small changes in their thinking and behavior every day. Dr. Dobson guides you each step of the way."
—Judith S. Beck, PhD, President,
Beck Institute for Cognitive Behavior Therapy

"Whether you are addressing your shyness and social anxiety for the first time, or want to keep making progress following treatment, this is a super resource! This book helps you identify how social anxiety is getting in your way and what you can do to interrupt the cycle. In an encouraging and optimistic tone, Dr. Dobson digs into the nitty-gritty of making friends, developing romantic relationships, and navigating the workplace, offering specific, practical tips aimed at helping you live your best life."
—Deborah Roth Ledley, PhD,
private practice, Philadelphia

"Packed with dozens of straightforward and practical strategies that target core elements of social anxiety. Dr. Dobson helps you gain new insights into your anxiety experiences and learn innovative ways of coping. Most important, this book shows how you can build richer social connections to reduce loneliness and boost life satisfaction."
—David A. Clark, PhD, coauthor
of *The Anxiety and Worry Workbook*

"Simply wonderful—one of the most helpful self-help books I have seen! If you are a therapist, you will want your clients with social anxiety to try out the skills in this book."
—Nina Josefowitz, PhD,
private practice, Toronto, Ontario, Canada

THE GUILFORD LIVING WELL SERIES

The Guilford Living Well Series is designed to help individuals with common psychological conditions solve everyday problems and optimize their quality of life. Readers get specific, empathic advice for stress-proofing daily routines; navigating work, family, and relationship issues; managing symptoms effectively; and finding answers to treatment questions. Written by leading experts on each disorder, books in the series are concise, practical, and empowering.

Living Well with Bipolar Disorder
David J. Miklowitz

Living Well with OCD
Jonathan S. Abramowitz

Living Well with Psychosis
Aaron P. Brinen

Living Well with Adult ADHD
Laura E. Knouse and Russell A. Barkley

Living Well with Social Anxiety
Deborah Dobson

FORTHCOMING

Living Well with Depression
Christopher R. Martell

living well *with*

social anxiety

PRACTICAL STRATEGIES
FOR IMPROVING YOUR DAILY LIFE

DEBORAH DOBSON, PhD

gp

THE GUILFORD PRESS

NEW YORK　LONDON

Printed in the United States of America

For product and safety concerns within the EU, please contact *GPSR@taylorandfrancis.com,* Taylor & Francis Verlag GmbH, Kaufingerstraße 24, 80331 München, Germany.

Last digit is print number: 9   8   7   6   5   4   3   2   1

This publication is intended to provide helpful and informative material. It is not intended to diagnose, treat, cure, or prevent any health problem or condition, nor is it intended to replace the advice of a health professional. No action should be taken based solely on the contents of this book. Always consult your physician or qualified health care professional on any matters regarding your health and before adopting any suggestions in this book or drawing inferences from it.

The author and publisher specifically disclaim all responsibility for any liability, loss, or risk, personal or otherwise, which is incurred as a consequence, directly or indirectly, from the use or application of any contents of this book.

Any and all product names referenced within this book are the trademarks of their respective owners. Always read all information provided by the manufacturers' product labels before using their products. The author and publisher are not responsible for claims made by manufacturers.

Library of Congress Cataloging-in-Publication Data is available from the publisher.

ISBN 978-1-4625-5425-6 (paperback)   ISBN 978-1-4625-5857-5 (hardcover)

contents

PART THREE
Living Your Best Life

acknowledgments

The opportunity to write this book came at a good time, as I was already reflecting on my years of work with people with social anxiety disorder. I had stepped back from my clinical work and was looking for ways to continue to contribute to the field. Writing this book has allowed me to think about the problems and ongoing effects and struggles that may continue for people with mental disorders despite treatment. I have thought about the many people who have influenced and inspired my work. This book would not have been possible without the support of many people, including colleagues, students, friends, family, and clients.

I have been very fortunate to have worked with many thoughtful and brilliant people and have enjoyed these collaborations tremendously. Throughout the years that I developed and conducted individual and group therapy for people with social anxiety, some of my major influences have been (in no particular order) Cherie Peterson, Jennifer Garinger-Orwin, Barb Backs-Dermott, Kerry Mothersill, Gayle Belsher, Nina Josefowitz, James Nieuwenhuis, Doug Watson, Jane Aldous, Dana McDougall, Caelin White, Michael Enman, David Hodgins, Roslyn Mendelson, and Candace Konnert. It has been a privilege to have had many students as co-therapists who always have new ideas and refreshing insights. The staff and student cognitive-behavioral therapy consultation group that I attended for many years provided weekly inspiration, support, intellectual challenges, and friendships. Thank you for all of those good times.

I would like to thank The Guilford Press and its editorial staff and consultants, most notably Christine Benton and Kitty Moore, for their support and guidance. Writing a book that is geared not for an academic or clinical audience but for the public was a very different experience for me and one that I could not have done without Christine and Kitty's expert guidance, patience, and feedback. It was not only a privilege to work with the two of you but also lots of fun! I looked forward to sitting down and writing and doing revisions, which is not something I was able to say about most projects that I've worked on.

My partner in life, Keith Dobson, encouraged me to take on this project and provided support every step of the way. He read the chapters and provided lots of feedback, and without him in the background I likely would not have found it possible to complete the book. I would also like to acknowledge the ongoing love and support from our children, Kit and Beth, their partners, Aubrey and Simon, and our grandchildren, Alex, Clem, Emma, and Thomas. Different perspectives and a few laughs along the way helped the ideas flow.

Many, many people experience social anxiety. I have worked with clients who have these struggles, and my life has been touched deeply by them. Writing about most of the strategies in this book led me to think of the times when I utilized them with clients and modified them with expert feedback from those with lived experiences. I hope that this book will contribute and provide ideas for those who are trying to improve and live their best lives.

living well with social anxiety

introduction

Social anxiety is a very common problem that affects many people. I imagine you picked up this book for one of the following reasons:

- You have been diagnosed as having social anxiety, and may have had treatment for it.
- You suspect you have this problem and are hoping there are things you can do on your own to help you with it.
- You're shy and feel frustrated because you'd like to enjoy being around people rather than feeling anxious.
- You would like to improve your coping and social skills.

Social anxiety can range from mild and specific to severe, disabling, and generalized, but there are lots of strategies you can use to live a richer life. This book is for you if you have any type of social anxiety, are shy, or are very socially isolated and want to be more connected to other people. While information is helpful, a great deal can be said for action. This book is focused on helping you learn and do something new to change.

Read on if you:

- worry that others are judging you negatively.
- say yes to requests from others when you want to say no.

- turn down interesting opportunities because they involve challenges such as making presentations to a group.
- rehash what you've said at gatherings or agonize over the impression you've made.
- keep your opinions to yourself—no matter how strongly you feel about them—when you believe others will disagree.
- curtail your activities, restrict your goals, and limit your life in other ways because of social anxiety.
- have been treated for social anxiety and continue to struggle with avoidance.

Most of us can relate to at least some of these concerns, and almost everyone has worried about either their effect on others or how they are viewed. It's normal to want to be liked and thought well of by others. It's common to be anxious in new situations, particularly when you know others are observing. If you experience social anxiety disorder, however, these thoughts can be overwhelming and have a huge impact on your life.

I was drawn to write this book because all of us want to live our best lives and to live well with whatever conditions, differences, illnesses, or disadvantages we have. We all have some type of disability just like we all have many abilities. I have worn glasses for nearsightedness and astigmatism since I was seven years old. I recently started wearing hearing aids. I have to adapt to these sensory aids and remember to use them. I am very short and cannot see much in a crowd of people except for the few people directly in front of me. While this is not a disability, it requires adaptation in an increasingly tall world!

At least one in five people will experience a mental health problem in any given year, and many of these 20% will have more than one diagnosis. If you have social anxiety to any degree, you have lots of company! Just like you, many others need information and strategies to live as best they can. Just like you, they have to use the help available to them so they can live the way they want to live.

If you've been treated for social anxiety disorder, you may know that the typical treatments are cognitive-behavioral therapy (CBT), provided either one on one or in a group setting, and/or medications. It can be challenging to access effective treatments—you may have tried and had to wait for a long time. If you've been fortunate enough to be able to access treatment, it may have been very helpful to you. Treatment has been shown repeatedly to reduce distress, improve understanding, provide skills, and change the way you view yourself as well as how you handle challenging situations. Treatment is in fact integral to recovery for many people. It also helps reduce or eliminate secondary problems, such as avoidance or the overuse of medications to manage anxiety.

Even if treatment helped and left you feeling much better, however, it's not the entire answer. It's likely that your social anxiety has not disappeared completely. You may continue to struggle with avoidance of social situations. It's common to keep having difficulties in some situations, and you may fall back into old patterns during life transitions or times of stress. The temptation to avoid situations to reduce anxiety can be overwhelming. So it's important to learn to both accept and challenge patterns of thinking and actions that go along with them. Most people find that problems are not permanently "cured" by treatment but occasionally recur. You will need to work to maintain gains made during therapy. It is extremely helpful to learn strategies to live well and take charge of social anxiety.

This book is intended to help you live well alongside social anxiety whether you're reading about the problem for the first time or trying to maintain gains following treatment. Social anxiety tends to be a long-lasting condition that begins during adolescence. I do not use the word *chronic*, though, because unlike chronic conditions such as some types of depression, some of the features of social anxiety are an integral part of who you are. For many people, the problem is long-term and could be considered a "trait" rather than a temporary "state." Most people who are shy are extremely sensitive to their social environment, and that can be a very positive feature. If you are introverted and care deeply about others, that is part of your character. Tempering extreme sensitivity can be helpful, but the world also needs sensitive, caring, and vulnerable people.

I have been a psychologist all of my career and have provided CBT to hundreds, if not thousands, of people with social anxiety. (I've never counted!) I have been humbled and honored to work with people who struggle but manage to thrive. I have been surprised at their resilience, creativity, and resourcefulness. People who work hard generally do well, and yet they may continue to have residual symptoms and vulnerabilities. It's certainly not fair, but it's true! Overall, it takes time, persistence, and effort to live well with social anxiety, but it will pay off. Treatments work, but ongoing strategies can help you live your best life before, during, and after therapy. This book is filled with strategies you can experiment with in different types of social situations to create and maintain change.

This book is not intended to replace treatment. It is, however, based on evidence-based strategies that follow the same principles and are consistent with CBT. You can read it from start to finish or pick it up when you want some new ideas. You'll read about people with similar struggles who have used various ideas, actions, and strategies to live well with social anxiety. I hope they will inspire you to do the same. All of the vignettes in this book are completely fictional—they are composites of different people that I've known over my years of talking to those with social anxiety.

This book is divided into three main sections, starting with a more general exploration of how social anxiety affects you and becoming more and more specific in terms of strategies for everyday situations. Part One, Taking Charge of Social Anxiety, is intended to help you understand social anxiety and the consequences that it has for your life. You will learn how to sort out the differences between your emotions, reactions, and thoughts. Once you pinpoint the problems, you will feel a greater sense of control over anxiety rather than feel like a puppet controlled by your fears. You will learn how to set goals for change that are consistent with your values and that are practical and useful. While you already know that social anxiety restricts your life, you will start to see the path forward. When you commit to change and begin to develop tools, the path to the future opens up.

Part Two, Daily-Life Strategies for Change in Social Anxiety, focuses on the three main interrelated components that will help lead to change: your physiological reactions and emotions; the thoughts that are at the root of your difficulties; and your behavioral reactions, particularly avoidance and exposure to situations that are scary for you. You will learn how to challenge yourself when anticipating worst-case scenarios that lead to avoidance. Because of long-term patterns and reactions, the urge to avoid can feel overwhelming, but obeying the urge perpetuates the problem. It is common to do things that you believe are helpful but seriously undermine your progress. Avoidance is the enemy of progress, and Part Two offers many strategies to help you "avoid avoidance." It will help you assess your reactions and understand what to do to challenge them. Breaking the cycle of social anxiety involves responding differently and engaging in difficult but enriching activities that build confidence over time.

Part Three, Living Your Best Life, turns to the development of skills and the courage to form connections with other people. Many people who are socially anxious have good social skills but struggle to use them or to put themselves in situations where they can try. Examples include basic skills for initiating conversations, meeting people, and starting to make friends. Part Three will cover more complex skills such as those needed for job interviews, presentations, and managing conflict. What constitutes "good social skills" is subjective, and there are lots of opinions about the best way to go about forming and maintaining relationships. The key is usually to have the courage to try, to give yourself permission to make and learn from your mistakes, and the resilience to try again. The problems and solutions presented in these chapters will help loosen the grip that social anxiety has on you and put you in charge of your life. The final chapter will look to the future and respond to the question of how to maintain change and continue to grow in your life.

Ultimately, this is a book about hope and optimism. Many people struggle silently with social anxiety, longing for the rich life among others that they deserve. The following pages will help you adopt the mindset and build the skills you need to rob social anxiety of its power over your life and go where you want to go.

PART ONE

taking charge
of social anxiety

1

how is social anxiety limiting your life?

Jody thinks of herself as shy. At 31, she has often felt lonely, and that's only getting worse now that she's moved to a new city for a job transfer and knows almost no one. She wants to prove herself in her new position, so she takes on extra tasks to show she's a hard worker. She'd like to date but finds the prospect terrifying, so she puts it off and tells herself she can't fit it in anyway, considering her long hours. Longtime low self-esteem also tells her she doesn't measure up to other women in this city who seem sophisticated and confident.

Ryan is 20 and has been reclusive since the beginning of the COVID-19 pandemic. He's extremely isolated, lacks life skills and experience, and avoids social contact. Now he feels depressed and irritable. His only social connections are through the gaming world. He lives in his parents' basement and plays online games most of the night. He either avoids thinking about the future or has impractical plans, such as developing gaming software. When he is forced to be out in public during the day, he avoids eye contact, wears a baseball cap and hoodie, and deliberately looks grouchy so that others don't approach him.

Jorge, 38 and single, has a good job in information technology and has a close family. He thinks of himself as outgoing, and yet his life is limited by a closely guarded secret and the machinations he goes through to keep it

hidden: He is terrified of public speaking. He hates being the center of atten-
tion in formal, structured situations and has become a master of excuses that
get him out of them. He responds rather than initiates, prepares extensively,
and hesitates to speak up in groups. Declined opportunities for advancement
have limited his career. And now his fear of public speaking is threatening
his social life too. A few months ago, a cousin asked him to give a toast at
an upcoming wedding, and he reluctantly accepted despite his private terror.
He's trying to come up with a good excuse to bow out but is feeling sad and
guilty about letting down his cousin and disappointing himself.

How is social anxiety limiting your life? Are the issues faced by Jody, Ryan, or Jorge similar to those that you face? I'm guessing that you will see parts of yourself in many of the examples in this book and that this will lead to insights and ways to reduce the restrictions on your life.

These three people appear to be very different from each other but have some core similarities in that they all struggle with social anxiety. They all avoid social situations in ways that are obvious or subtle. Jody hesitates to speak up and say no to unwanted tasks and to take steps to initiate friendships, whereas Ryan avoids in-person interactions and making long-term decisions. While Jorge is comfortable in casual situations, he has a fear of speaking in front of a group. Social anxiety has many faces, from mild discomfort in some situations or intense fear in specific social situations, to severe and disabling fear and avoidance. All of these fears place limits on life.

Avoiding Discomfort: A Slippery Slope

Avoidance of difficult or challenging situations is key to keeping social anxiety alive and well. It has become quite easy and seems quite normal in many parts of the world to use digital technology for tasks that previously required us to show up in person. Not everyone has access to technology, but many of us can do most of our day-to-day activities without having an in-person conversation. Does this feel comfortable to you? Avoidance of in-person contact may seem preferable, but it becomes a risky habit.

The pandemic of the early 2020s damaged mental health in many ways. A major cause of emotional suffering since then has been the continued lack of in-person social contact. Many of us underestimated the importance of everyday contact such as being in line at a coffee shop or saying hello to a receptionist at an office. We may never have thought about the fact that even being in the presence of others without talking is helpful, as it reminds us that we are part of a larger community. During lockdown, we had to find new ways to interact with other people, and we got very creative, using digital technology to have virtual meetings and parties, playing new types of games online, and more. Now we are comfortable with ordering our meals, managing our finances, and keeping in touch with people without seeing them face to face. We have contacts around the world that we have never met in person. Many people work remotely.

If you are socially anxious, this situation is a blessing and a curse. You probably both crave and fear interactions, believing you'll be judged or embarrassed or will come across negatively, yet wanting the human contact we all need. When the social distancing of the pandemic eased, many people commented that they felt uncomfortable in crowds and in loud places and that their social skills were "rusty" due to lack of practice. Those with social anxiety may have become even more comfortable avoiding social contact than they were before the pandemic. Unfortunately, the short-term ease of social avoidance takes its toll over the longer term. It is very natural and easy to avoid what is difficult—we all do it—but what do we lose in exchange? Our lives are limited by this avoidance.

Think of five tasks that you don't do in person anymore but have in the recent past. For me, they include shopping, buying tickets for events, ordering food from restaurants, taking a course, and attending meetings. Write yours in the spaces below or outside this book.

Five Tasks I Complete Online

1. _____

2. _____

3. _____

4. _____

5. _____

While some of these tasks have an interpersonal component, such as online meetings, they don't involve face-to-face interaction. If you live alone and work from home, it's easy to go for days without seeing another person. Consider the loss of social connection and practice involved and it's easy to see why social anxiety becomes worsened with lack of contact with others. It's far easier to lose contact and maintain that loss than it is to reconstruct a social life. It takes understanding, effort, and consistent practice to make changes.

Now consider the past few days. How many people have you encountered? Did you speak to them? Did you do a task that involved interacting with another person? If a socially anxious person has low rates of social interaction and it is more convenient to avoid rather than engage with others, problems will become worse. It will be impossible for Ryan to recover if he continues to avoid people. Jody will not magically start to meet people if she continues to stay at work after hours completing tasks that no one else wants to do.

> Avoidance is a big problem, and the solution is to minimize it as much as possible.

What Does Your Social Anxiety Look Like?

People who are socially anxious go out of their way to avoid feeling uncomfortable. So how does it feel to be socially anxious? How does social anxiety show up in your thoughts and your behavior? Making changes to live better with social anxiety depends on understanding all the ways in which anxiety is affecting you, so it's important to take a close look at it.

While you are likely very familiar with many of the signs of social anxiety, there may be symptoms that you have not recognized in yourself. Identifying these signs is like taking them apart one by one and looking at them in the daylight. By doing this, you can help demystify them. Understanding your symptoms can help you tackle them. A formal diagnosis takes time and a comprehensive interview by a mental health professional, but the following questions can give you an idea of how social anxiety takes shape in your life.

How Does Your Social Anxiety Take Shape?

❑ Do you often worry about what others think about you?

❑ Do you think they may judge you in a negative way?

❑ Do you fear that you will embarrass yourself in front of others?

❑ Do you avoid some or most social interactions?

❑ Do you dislike being the center of attention, such as when you are reading aloud?

❑ Do you tend to wait for others to approach you rather than initiate conversations yourself?

❑ Do you show visible signs of anxiety, such as sweating, blushing, or trembling?

❑ Does your anxiety ever happen "all of a sudden" with intense physical signs such as a very dry mouth or racing heart?

Your answers to these questions will give you clues to which problems to address first. No doubt, you worry about what other people think about you, as virtually everyone with social anxiety does. But you can focus on learning skills for challenging your anxious thoughts. If you avoid initiating conversations, you can learn skills to take the first step in talking to others. If you dislike being the center of attention, you can learn to tolerate the fact that others do notice you but probably not as much as you think. It's important to learn ways to accept being visible as well as to learn from observing other people.

Is Your Social Anxiety General or Specific?

❑ Do you worry about most or all social situations?

❑ Do you fear just a few specific social situations, such as dating or putting yourself in vulnerable positions like letting someone know you're interested in a friendship?

❑ Do you fear being observed doing something specific such as signing your name, eating in front of others, or engaging in a sport?

❑ Do you fear public speaking?

Your answers to these questions deepen your understanding of the scope of your social anxiety. If you answered yes to the first question, your anxiety is broad and its impact greater on your overall life. While most people with generalized social anxiety are also afraid of public speaking, they often don't fear being observed doing something specific.

Specific social anxiety is more focused, but still can be a major problem. It can vary from fear of signing one's name or writing while being observed to urinating in public washrooms (for biological males) or performing an act such as dancing while being watched. If you fear eating or drinking in front of others, for example, you likely spend a great deal of time planning, avoiding, and restricting your life to limit public exposure of your eating and drinking. Food and drink are an important part of most social events. People with performance fears, such as eating, drinking, dancing, or doing an activity while being observed, dislike being the center of attention and worry about making mistakes (like spilling, making a mess, or stumbling) and becoming embarrassed.

Learning skills to engage in your feared situations rather than avoid them can be very freeing but it can be scary to go through the process. Change involves calculated risks. You can learn many ways to plan small, deliberate risks and develop confidence as you take these steps.

You're Not as Alone as You Think

Most people who are socially anxious feel different and alone. Avoidance feeds on itself. It also makes us feel more alone than we are. Take a look at the chart on page 15. As you can see, social anxiety is common and shyness is even more common. Social anxiety affects over 10% of the population over their lifetimes. About 40% of adults label themselves as shy—that's almost half the adult population!

RATES OF SOCIAL ANXIETY IN NORTH AMERICA

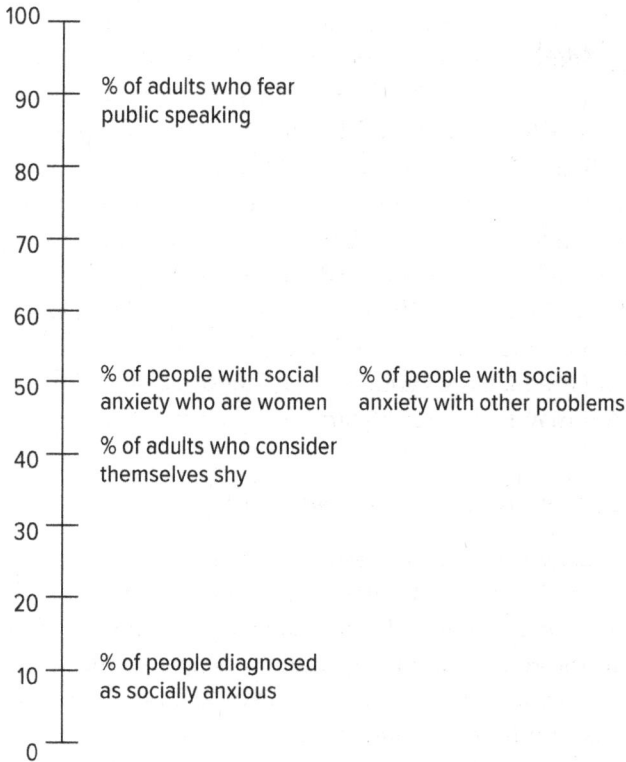

```
100 ┬
    │
 90 ┼  % of adults who fear
    │  public speaking
 80 ┼
    │
 70 ┼
    │
 60 ┼
    │
 50 ┼  % of people with social    % of people with social
    │  anxiety who are women      anxiety with other problems
 40 ┼  % of adults who consider
    │  themselves shy
 30 ┼
    │
 20 ┼
    │
 10 ┼  % of people diagnosed
    │  as socially anxious
  0 ┴
```

Shyness is not a mental health problem but an aspect of one's personality. Some people are more introverted and value being alone more than others. Social anxiety disorder is a mental health problem, and it usually does not go away on its own, unless something significant about the person's situation changes. (You may have heard the terms *social phobia, socially avoidant personality,* and *social anxiety disorder.* Social anxiety disorder is the term used in the *Diagnostic and Statistical Manual of Mental Disorders, Fifth Edition, Text Revision* [DSM-5-TR], which is used throughout much of the world.) The good news is that treatments work and there are lots of effective strategies to help people with these difficulties live their best lives. All of the strategies presented in this book are based on findings from evidence-based practice and research.

YOUR ANXIETY DOESN'T MAKE YOU STAND OUT

Observe the people around you and try to figure out how they might be feeling. Someone else may be even more anxious than you are. You might find this hard to believe. Spending a lot of time alone, avoiding others, can reinforce the false belief that others see right through you and can tell that you are anxious—another negative consequence of avoidance. In reality your anxiety is usually not obvious to others. If you're like others who are socially anxious—like Jody and Ryan—you are quiet and avoid contact. Your demeanor and your behavior can hide your anxiety. Many socially anxious people have told me they work hard to be invisible and not stand out in a crowd. Men and women are affected about equally, so you can't be identified as socially anxious by gender. You may be less visibly anxious than you think!

> **PRACTICE EXERCISE: Do a head count**
>
> Imagine that you are in a room of people and do a careful count of how many are present. Calculate 10% of the group, representing the percentage of the general population who are socially anxious. If there are 20 people in the room, how many anxious people would there be? Contrary to what you may believe, there can be comfort (and safety) in numbers. Look around the room and try to determine who else might be uncomfortable in addition to you. Now visualize approaching them as they stand on the sidelines and don't have anyone to talk to. They might appreciate having someone to talk to—you. It's difficult to know if they are anxious or not by observing, but you may pick up some clues from their actions. This experiment takes your attention away from yourself and focuses it on other people.

SOCIAL ANXIETY VARIES WIDELY IN SEVERITY

Clinicians and researchers think of social anxiety as being on a continuum from mild to severe. Variations in the symptoms of social anxiety make it difficult for others to identify you at a glance as being socially anxious. There's no single level of severity for all, and you may notice that your anxiety varies considerably across situations. The continuum ranges from shyness (again, not a mental disorder) to avoidant personality disorder, which tends to be a more disabling, chronic problem.

Social anxiety disorder is in the middle of that continuum. Milder forms of social anxiety can include fears of a few social situations. Most people with milder problems have some challenges but manage most of their required activities.

While fear of public speaking is not necessarily a problem if you are not expected to talk in front of others, it can create obstacles in certain lines of work (such as teaching) or in some situations, such as Jorge's. Approximately 90% of people say they are afraid of public speaking, so the 10% who are not fearful are clearly in the minority. When Jorge is giving his toast, many in the audience will be relieved that they weren't asked! He can also think of this statistic and be aware that many others share his fears.

Where Is Social Anxiety Interfering?

Even if your anxiety is mild, it can have far-ranging consequences and have a significant effect on your life. The following questions can reveal the impact of your social anxiety on your life as well as some of the other problems it has led to. You may then see where you can start to make some changes.

❑ Do you feel isolated, with fewer friendships and other relationships than you'd like?

❑ Do you wish you could feel more at ease around people and have a richer social life?

❑ Have you declined opportunities that you are interested in because of anxiety?

❑ Do you feel sad and lonely?

❑ Does anxiety linger and affect you most of the time, even when you're just thinking of something social?

❑ Have you ever not taken a class or job because you suspected there would be a presentation component?

❑ Have there been other negative consequences of social anxiety for you, such as becoming depressed or having panic attacks?

❑ Have you tried to reduce your anxiety with drugs or alcohol? Do you sometimes take a drink or a pill before an important social activity?

If you answered yes to many of these questions, you're beginning to see how limiting social anxiety can be, whether it's general or specific. Jorge felt bad about considering backing out of the wedding toast for his cousin, and he also began to see how his fears of speaking up were limiting his career advancement. He was concerned when he realized that he might be tempted to have a drink before the toast to "relax," and questioned how far he might take that strategy in other parts of his life.

Maybe answering these questions has led you to realize that your fears center on what you care most about. If you are fearful of being observed while playing tennis, it might not be a big deal if you only play for fun on weekends, but what if you are a competitive athlete and tennis matters tremendously to you? Conversely, if you don't care much about social connections with others, you would not likely be socially anxious. *For must of us, what matters most is what makes us most anxious.* Being anxious about what other people think means that you care.

Social anxiety can not only obstruct your most important goals by isolating you and leading you away from significant opportunities but it can also lead to serious consequences such as substance abuse, panic attacks, or depression. The good news is that there is a great deal that you can do to live well alongside the anxiety and live your best life. An important first step is understanding yourself and how your anxiety works. It is crucial to take charge of anxiety rather than allowing the anxiety to order you around. You want to be the boss, and there is a great deal that you can do about social anxiety.

All of Life Is a Stage: The Key Feature of Social Anxiety

A client once told me that they felt as though all social situations were like performances on a life stage. It was like the theater critics were all sitting in the audience. When on stage, it is easy to be anxious! In such situations, you may make negative predictions that your mind will go blank, that you will say the wrong thing, appear "stupid," or make a social gaffe. Everything will stop and people will stare.

Because of these thoughts, you will feel extremely self-conscious and scrutinize yourself very closely. If you are carefully observing yourself, you won't be observing others very well and will feel more anxious. There is only so much attention to go around, and if your focus is on yourself, there is not much left over to observe others and learn about the situation. If life seems like a performance, think of the rehearsal, energy, and worry demanded by anxiety. There is not much room left for spontaneity and enjoyment, and normal life is limited. The point of change is to focus less on potential mistakes and more on just living life well.

Since the key feature of social anxiety is a fear of being embarrassed in public or negatively evaluated by other people, becoming aware of and changing these thoughts is a big part of the solution. Social anxiety and performance anxiety are essentially the same thing.

Is It People or Performance That Makes You Anxious?

Jody worries that she is not accepted or liked by her coworkers and would not fit in at their annual fall party. Jorge has anticipatory thoughts that he will stutter over his words and his mind will go completely blank during his toast. Ryan is convinced that there is no one else in the world outside of the online community that he could relate to and who would accept him. For these three people, these thoughts lead to avoidance of exactly the situation that could open up their lives. For Jody this is meeting others in a casual setting and perhaps making friends. For Jorge it is celebrating his cousin by giving the toast and feeling proud of himself. For Ryan it is meeting a peer in person and realizing that they have commonalities and could perhaps even become friends.

Consider how your worry about social situations limits your life. These thoughts can be very distracting and lead to exactly the things they predict. Jorge might worry so much that he actually does stutter and lose his place in the speech. If you were an actor, you'd have to learn how to manage these negative thoughts as well as get past the occasional mistake. A very important part of change is learning how to harness these thoughts and rein them in. Thoughts affect what you do and how you behave. Perhaps you've heard the saying "Dance as though no one is watching." This statement means to perform with joy and without embarrassment.

> Negative predictions lead to avoidance,
> and challenging them is key to change.

How Does Performance Anxiety Take Up Space in Your Mind?

Social fears typically occur in your thoughts before, during, and following social interactions. If you see others daily—and I hope you do—these fears can take up a great deal of mental space.

ANXIETY BEFORE A SOCIAL EVENT

The greatest intensity of fear tends to be in advance of a social event, sometimes lasting for days or weeks and peaking shortly before the event. Anticipatory anxiety can lead to excessive planning, making negative predictions, or just plain avoidance. It's easy to talk yourself out of things and make excuses because of anxiety. Some planning is helpful: What will I wear? What are some topics that I could talk about? Who could I talk to? Where is the event? But trying to plan conversations in detail is bound to fail, as others are not predictable and conversations lead in all sorts of directions. Later in this book I offer practical suggestions for dealing with conversations with less social anxiety.

ANXIETY DURING A SOCIAL EVENT

Often fears decrease once the event has begun and you realize that it's not as terrible as you expected. Heightened self-observation, though, certainly can and does occur throughout events and can be very inhibiting. Many anxious people are quite quiet, may avoid eye contact, and try to be invisible. For example, if Jody went to the work party, she might stand to the side, wait for others to approach her, and leave early. Jorge might ask to be the first person to give a speech and try to get through his toast as quickly as possible, hoping that his talk will be forgotten as the others will be more interesting and entertaining. Many people who are socially anxious have lots of different strategies to manage their anxiety, many of which involve avoidance such as trying to blend into the crowd. During the event, anxiety is likely to go up and down, depending on what is happening and your thoughts about it. For example, if introductions are occurring and your turn is coming up, anxiety is likely to rise and then fall after it's over.

ANXIETY AFTER A SOCIAL EVENT

Following an event, you may have noticed that you sometimes review what occurred in detail and become more anxious or even angry at yourself for what you said or didn't say. We've all had the experience of thinking of the best response after the fact! You may ruminate about something you said for a long time, and yet if you get up the nerve to ask someone else about it, they might not even remember what you said. Jody might berate herself for how she thinks she came across to others. Jorge will likely compare his toast to others and may be self-critical, while also being pleased that he gave it. Have you ever worried for days about a perceived social faux pas, finally asked a friend about it, and found they had no idea what you were talking about? The fear of negative evaluation leads to thoughts that others are more judgmental than they actually are. Our perceived mistakes often go unnoticed by other people.

> Think of how much mental real estate would be freed up in your mind if you had fewer worries before, during, and after social events occur.

What Are Your Physical Signs of Anxiety?

Physical signs of anxiety are common, especially just before or during an event. These may include heart palpitations, faster breathing, sweating, blushing, or trembling. Socially anxious people tend to blush more than the average person, which has always struck me as unfair, as it is one of the few visible signs of anxiety. Other signs can include a dry mouth, which can make it difficult to talk. When you are highly anxious, it can even be difficult to think or remember.

A panic attack is a sudden rush of fear, usually accompanied by intense physical symptoms such as a pounding heart, feelings of dizziness or faintness, and a sense of unreality. Panic attacks brought on by social anxiety can and do occur, and can feel very uncomfortable although they are not usually visible to others.

As anxiety takes energy, it is common to feel tired after social events. When you're anxious, your body becomes super-alert and full of adrenaline, which uses up a lot of energy. That explains why you're so tired after spending time in social situations. Following the pandemic, many people noticed that they were more fatigued after being around groups of people—that is because their anxiety systems were working harder than when they were alone.

You may have noticed having strong reactions when you've been nervous and not known how to interpret them. Our body has a physical response to anxiety that may be interpreted by our mind in different ways. At times these responses can lead to irritability or even anger. You don't want to attract attention from other people, so you may look away or scowl at them. Ryan often works hard to keep others at a distance, which is fairly common for people who are socially anxious.

These physical reactions are uncomfortable and sometimes confusing, but they're not dangerous. It can feel difficult to push through them, but you'll find that it's worth the effort.

The Cost of Staying in Your Comfort Zone

It's easier to be comfortable than it is to be anxious. This is why we allow social anxiety to dictate how we live our lives. Negative predictions, thoughts, and fears lead to different types of avoidance, which is completely understandable under the circumstances. Why would you do something that is terrifying and uncomfortable, and that you predict will go very badly? People who are socially anxious may avoid social interactions completely, have a limited comfort zone, or suffer through things with great difficulty. You may be a master of excuses, made either to yourself or to others.

Do you ever find yourself being quite gregarious in social situations, speaking very quickly, being intolerant of natural silences in conversations, asking many questions and yet avoiding talking about yourself? This is a social anxiety cover-up. You take refuge in controlling the conversation to avoid the discomfort of leaving yourself vulnerable to judgment. Chattering can feel like a good way to avoid others' controlling the situation. That way, you may not have to answer questions about yourself and can focus on the other people.

Social anxiety can take surprising forms. Do you avoid sharing your opinions out of fear that they will be viewed as wrong or stupid? This can look like humility or courtesy, but it's also another social anxiety mask. Maybe you come across as irritable, standoffish, or even angry. Many people with social anxiety have told me that others have viewed them as unfriendly or snobbish. Yet another social anxiety ruse. It's an effective way to push people away.

Consider how these tendencies keep you in your comfort zone and limit your life. If you don't share your opinions, others will not know what they are and you'll be misunderstood. If you don't share your preferences, even about small things, you won't get what you want or need. Getting out of your comfort zone is scary and will feel risky, but it will get you on the path to change.

Starting Something Is Harder Than Sticking with It

Unsurprisingly, starting to date or interviewing for a job exposes you to some judgment. The fact that you don't know in advance whether the verdict will be positive or negative calls up social anxiety. So you probably find starting relationships more difficult than maintaining them or being in a job easier than interviewing for one. Clients have told me that if they could get a job without an interview, they probably would be fine; it's the initial part of putting themselves out there that is so difficult. When beginning something new, it's obvious that some judgment, either positive, negative, or neutral, is occurring. It's important to learn strategies to realistically assess and tolerate the evaluation that occurs at the beginning of any new venture, be it a relationship, school, or job.

Counting the Consequences

You now have an idea of the scope of your social anxiety. You know whether it permeates your life or focuses on one fear that imposes pervasive limitations on how you conduct your life. You've become familiar with how often you feel like your whole life is a performance—one that will invariably earn you a terrible review from your imagined audience. You've taken a closer look at how social anxiety invades your thoughts, produces physical discomfort, and leads to isolating, avoidant behavior. Now it's time to take stock of the consequences. Looking squarely at how social anxiety has kept you from living well can motivate you to push your way out of your comfort zone and into the life you really want. It may be painful to self-reflect this deeply, but see if you can honestly unveil the damage social anxiety is doing to your life by checking off which of the following you have experienced:

❑ Low self-esteem and feeling unworthy

❑ Self-criticism and harsh self-judgment

❑ Anticipation of the worst outcomes for yourself, so opportunities are lost and invitations declined (and may eventually fade away)

❑ Interference in career and educational goals (reported by over 80% of people with social anxiety in surveys)

❑ Relationships formed less often and less easily

Additional Consequences—More Mental Health Problems

Over half of the people with social anxiety develop other, secondary mental health problems (*secondary* meaning these problems develop because of the social anxiety), such as the following:

• **Substance abuse:** Higher rates of alcohol or drug use (in the name of "loosening up") leave people with social anxiety susceptible to developing a substance abuse problem. You may notice that you regularly have a drink or take an anti-anxiety medication before a social event that you are anxious about. It's easy to fall into the habit of doing this, and if you do you may develop a substance abuse problem over time and end up with two problems where you started with one. If you are concerned, don't hesitate to talk to your medical practitioner and have an assessment.

• **Other types of anxiety disorders:** Panic attacks, panic disorder with agoraphobia, and generalized anxiety disorder are all common among people with social anxiety. Some people will experience panic attacks in social situations, which can lead to further worry and anxiety about the panic. If the panic occurs only in social situations, these are part of the social anxiety disorder. How would you feel about shopping in a large mall if it were completely empty, but you could still make your purchases? If you have just social anxiety, you probably don't mind being in large open spaces where there is no risk of being observed and judged. If you wouldn't want to go to an empty mall, you might have panic disorder and agoraphobia rather than social anxiety because you fear not being able to access help in this situation, rather than being scrutinized. In reading this book, you will learn strategies to manage intense reactions such as panic attacks as well as being visible in public situations.

• **Depression:** Loneliness and isolation can lead to depression. Social connections are antidepressant in nature, and people thrive on interactions. I'm predicting that you are reading this book because you want to increase and improve your relationships with others. Being unable to complete school, work, or have relationships can be depressing! In fact, depression may have been a catalyst for you to seek help by reading this book. While the treatment strategies for social anxiety can also help with depression, it may be important to obtain additional help, especially if low mood prevents you from doing regular activities. Once you engage more in your life and learn skills to become more comfortable around people and feel less isolated, your mood will also start to improve.

• **Avoidant personality disorder:** At the extreme end of the social anxiety continuum lies avoidant personality disorder, which can be difficult to distinguish from severe social anxiety disorder. This is a chronic form of social anxiety with hypersensitivity to judgment, intense feelings of inadequacy, and inhibition. It tends to be long-lasting, and individuals with this problem live restrained and isolated lives. Because people with this diagnosis are expert avoiders, their exposure to social anxiety triggers is lower than for severe social anxiety disorder, and as a result they usually have fewer physical signs of anxiety. The psychological treatments are similar to those for social anxiety, and the strategies in this book are all applicable.

How Social Anxiety Develops

Most people with social anxiety were shy as children and may have grown up in families where others were shy as well. Typically, difficulties begin in adolescence and are more marked during times of transition, such as starting high school, beginning a relationship, moving away from home to college, or looking for a full-time job for the first time. You have probably noticed that demands and stresses are greater during changes in life.

Social expectations tend to increase as teens develop, and structured and supervised interactions tend to decrease. Your social life was organized primarily by your parents when you were a child, but as you grew up you formed new interests and friendships. As your social identity developed, you started to compare yourself to others.

If you were anxious in adolescence, you may have started to struggle then and became very self-conscious, feeling like you didn't measure up. You wanted to be distinct and also to fit in with your classmates. Fearing their judgment may have led to avoiding and minimizing contact with your peers. In turn, your self-confidence may have suffered. Avoidance robbed you of opportunities to practice and develop the social skills that many adults have gained through experience (a gap that may explain why fewer adults than children see themselves as shy).

For a small subset of people social anxiety develops secondary to another problem instead of the other way around. You might have been socially isolated during critical periods of your development and missed out on important social experiences. Examples include teenagers who were seriously physically or mentally ill and missed out on lengthy periods of school while recuperating at home or hospitalized; people experiencing extended periods of isolation due to, for example, debilitating long COVID or immunocompromised systems have fewer opportunities for social interaction. These teenagers may fully recover from whatever led to their isolation but may need help to develop the social skills they missed out on. Or you might have been home-schooled or taken courses online and so advanced academically but not socially. For example, Ryan completed his diploma online during school lockdown, so he did not engage in the complex social interactions that normally occur in high school. A great deal happens in and out of the classroom, and it takes time, practice, and social feedback to learn these skills.

Some people develop social anxiety as a result of being visibly different from the majority of the population; see the box below. Communication and social skills are important strategies to overcome social anxiety that developed early and led to isolation. Learning and developing confidence using social skills will make your life less limited.

Visible Differences and Social Anxiety

People who are part of a visibly obvious minority group are likely to fear judgment and discrimination. Imagine for a moment that you want to blend into the crowd and not be visible, but by virtue of your skin color, the clothes that you wear, or your religious symbols, it is not possible to do so. Many people in these situations would feel vulnerable and exposed and possibly socially anxious. People from gender minorities may also be more likely to be socially anxious, due to both heightened fear of being judged (based on what they may think are their obvious visible differences) and their actual increased risk of being judged or discriminated against. I have had transgender clients who were forced to wear clothes of the opposite sex as children and felt extremely self-conscious and humiliated while doing so. These experiences had led to considerable anxiety when these individuals were out in public.

How to View the Question of Cause

It's only natural to wonder how you got here—how you ended up feeling so limited by social anxiety that your life seems narrowed. Like most mental health problems, your social anxiety most likely came from a combination of factors. Anxiety tends to "run in families," so part of how you got here is likely to be genetic, particularly a tendency toward what is called *behavioral inhibition*. If you're inhibited, you're likely to take fewer risks, including social ones, and you may be quite reserved. You may observe carefully before doing things and be "slow to warm up" to others.

If you have parents and siblings with similar dispositions, the environment that you grew up in was likely quiet and had few social opportunities. You may have learned to be wary around others. Of course, it is difficult to separate "nature" from "nurture" as there are both genetic and environmental factors. We observe our parents and learn about social interactions from them. Many anxious people also have a greater sensitivity to anxiety, possibly creating more intense feelings of discomfort with physical signs of fear thus leading to avoidance.

Consequently, the causes are likely a combination of disposition, personality style, and experiences. You may be unable to remember a time when you did not feel anxious, whereas others clearly remember being carefree as a child and then becoming very self-conscious during adolescence. A considerable number of socially anxious people have a history of being bullied, teased, or humiliated, which plays a significant role in either the onset or the worsening of this problem. Unfortunately, children who appear shy and vulnerable may become targets of teasing.

Even though genetic factors, learning, and early experiences play important roles in causing anxiety, lots can be done to improve the current situation. That's because it's more important to consider what maintains anxiety in your daily life than what started that ball rolling. You can't change your genetics, disposition, or past experiences anyway, so why not turn to what you *can* control? You can certainly work on living well in the present. You can become aware of and work on factors that maintain anxiety. Maintenance factors are what keeps anxiety alive and gives it energy to keep going.

As noted early in this chapter, the single biggest maintenance factor is avoidance. When you avoid, you miss out on new experiences, cannot challenge your thoughts, and often convince yourself that avoidance is the best option. Avoidance and maintenance factors are discussed in detail in Chapter 6 to help cut off the fuel to your social anxiety.

On the Way to Change

It is important to consider that there are pros and cons to social anxiety. What are some of the positives for you of being socially anxious? For example, you may be sensitive to the emotions and needs of others, be emotionally intelligent, or be a very loyal friend and employee. These are all strengths to celebrate and build on. While reducing the negative aspects and limitations of having social anxiety, it's important to remember some of the positive attributes that make you who you are.

Understanding the context helps you on the way to change. I suspect that you have tried lots of things to manage your problems—ensure that you give yourself credit for different efforts to cope and build on those that have been helpful. These strategies may include reading about social anxiety, using relaxation strategies, or consulting mobile apps. These efforts show curiosity and a strong desire to improve your life and reduce the effects of anxiety.

Moving Forward

Social anxiety is part of you, but not all of you, and you can make it a smaller part. It doesn't have to define you. The understanding you've gained in this chapter about how social anxiety is limiting your life may have made you eager to get started on change. Taking charge is key. While others can provide information, suggestions, and ideas, you are the only one who can try them out and take the risk of making changes. Change cannot happen without some risk. Reducing social anxiety's grip on you cannot start without some discomfort. But it won't necessarily be a lot of discomfort. You have also found that observing others instead of yourself reduces your social anxiety a little bit all by itself—a nice incentive to start giving some thought to what you want to change to live well, the subject of the next chapter.

2

how can you interrupt the social anxiety cycle?

Chapter 1 helped you take a good look at how social anxiety is interfering with your life. Since you've gotten to this chapter, it must have reinforced your belief that it's wise to start taking charge of social anxiety and get on with living your best life. Now what?

You now have a working knowledge of how social anxiety operates. You certainly know how it feels! And you know that social anxiety takes different shapes for different people. You may have seen yourself in some of the people described in Chapter 1, who respond to social situations in some of the same ways that you do. But you may not have a clue about *why* you respond to social situations the way you do.

Understanding *why* is key to taking charge of your own social anxiety. Anxiety in general often elicits certain reactions before we even know what's happening. This chapter provides strategies for monitoring your own experiences with social anxiety so you know what's in play and can take advantage of opportunities to break what may seem like an impregnable cycle.

The Components of Social Anxiety: Thoughts, Feelings, and Actions

To break a cycle and understand why it happens, we need to identify its components. When you are anxious, your reactions happen quickly and tend to be a blur. Pushing pause to sort your reactions out and break the cycle down into its components will give you a sense of control.

Ten people in the same situation and will come away with ten different stories about it. We all interpret the world in different ways. These unique feelings and thoughts lead to different actions. You may have heard of or read about cognitive-behavioral therapy (CBT). If you have had CBT, it likely included learning about your thoughts, feelings, and actions and how to shift them so that you can feel better. While it is an oversimplification, psychologists talk about the cognitive behavioral triangle (see the diagram below) of thoughts—feelings—actions. How we feel both physically and emotionally affects how we think and what actions or inactions we take. Each of these points of the triangle affect the other two points, and it all takes place in the context of the situation.

> Lisa was on a work break during her job as a security guard at the mall. She went for a walk outside the building, as she tended to avoid people when she could. She had struggled with social anxiety for years. She felt uncomfortable and embarrassed when Jon, a colleague who she knew fairly well, did not respond to her greeting when walking down the street. Her first thought was that Jon must be angry at her, and she started thinking back to past events to figure out why. She hated it when anyone might be the least bit upset with her. Consequently, her **feeling** was discomfort, her **action** was

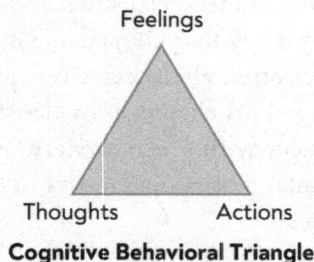

Feelings

Thoughts   Actions

Cognitive Behavioral Triangle

*first to say hi and then continue walking, and her **thought** was that Jon was angry. What she didn't see was that Jon turned around and waved at her as she walked away! It's easy to see how Lisa's first response (saying hello) initiated contact and how her thoughts led to her walking away and missing that Jon, distracted by his own thoughts, hadn't noticed her greeting right away. The next time Lisa encounters Jon, she might be hesitant and not say anything, leading him to feel confused and have thoughts of his own, such as "She is unfriendly." Given her worries about others becoming upset with her, Lisa is likely to be even more uncomfortable in this situation than someone who is not socially anxious.*

It's easy to see how Lisa's reaction led to certain follow-up actions or behaviors, which over time and left unchecked could influence her relationship with Jon. Misunderstandings are common and do not happen in a vacuum. They build on each other and exacerbate social anxiety.

Understanding through Self-Monitoring

One way to understand how thoughts, feelings, and actions work together to create social anxiety is self-monitoring. Monitoring is fairly easy in principle, but it takes time and practice to become proficient.

Jody attended a work party with her colleague Emily. They drove together in Emily's car and chatted about work on the way to the party, which helped Jody feel less anxious than she had felt while getting ready. Emily had a good sense of humor and after two years in the office knew many of their colleagues quite well, and provided the "inside scoop" on some upcoming changes that Jody had heard rumors about. Once they entered the door to the restaurant where the party was being held, Jody saw that the setting was formal—a sit-down dinner with assigned seats. This immediately threw her, and she became almost panicked as she saw that she wasn't seated with Emily. She was placed between two men who worked in the information technology department and across from one of the women whom she frequently saw laughing and talking in an animated way in the lunchroom. After checking her coat, she immediately went to the washroom as she felt as though she might throw up. She looked in the mirror and saw that her face was flushed and went into one of the stalls.

Jody's situation is a perfect example where self-monitoring could be used. Our responses tend to happen in a jumble, and we tend to react quickly before stopping to consider different options. We don't tend to naturally separate our feelings from our thoughts. Yet for each situation we encounter we can analyze our reactions and answer the following questions:

- What is the situation? (Where are you, who are you with, what is going on right now?)
- What is going through your mind? These thoughts—called your *automatic thoughts*—are your immediate internal commentary, and they come up without any planning. It can take practice to catch these thoughts before they disappear as quickly as they arose.
- What emotions are you experiencing? How intense are these feelings on a scale from 0 to 100? Think of this scale (shown below) as a kind of "feelings thermometer," with "no emotion at all" at 0 and the most intense emotion that you have ever felt at 100; you could also

EMOTIONAL INTENSITY SCALE FOR SOCIAL ANXIETY

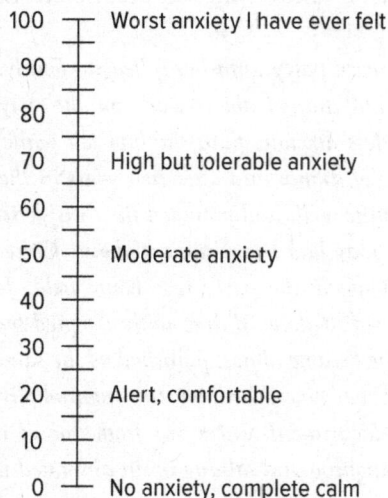

100	Worst anxiety I have ever felt
90	
80	
70	High but tolerable anxiety
60	
50	Moderate anxiety
40	
30	
20	Alert, comfortable
10	
0	No anxiety, complete calm

think of the intensity in terms of a percentage. (While the example provided here is anxiety, this scale can be used for any emotion, including those typically considered positive, such as excitement or joy.) Most of the time you will feel more than one emotion. Our gut reactions are the physical sensations that occur in our body and are directly related to these feelings.

- What are you doing? Sometimes, even more importantly, what are you not doing or maybe avoiding? Have you taken any actions to reduce or avoid your anxiety?

You can use the Thoughts, Feelings, and Actions Record on page 36 (also available to download and print and at *www.guilford.com/ dobson3-forms*) to enter this information. It takes self-awareness and practice to become skilled at self-monitoring, but once you learn how to do it it's a very useful strategy for all sorts of daily situations. It tends to work best if completed during or shortly following a situation, although doing it a few hours later works as well. I have placed the thoughts column prior to the feelings column whereas some similar charts have them the other way around. As they are very interconnected, it is impossible to know if thoughts lead to feelings or the reverse. It doesn't really matter!

Jody had encountered a thoughts, feelings, and actions worksheet in a book she had read about social anxiety, and once she was in the washroom she decided she would try to work through it on the thought record she had created on her phone. As she was in the stall, she had a comforting amount of privacy . . . although she knew that people often were on their phones, so no one would have had any idea what she was doing anyway. (If she were in a public place, she could pretend she was posting something on social media.)

The situation was straightforward to record—taking a break in the washroom stall while attending a work party at a formal restaurant. She was unsure what to record in the automatic thoughts column because quite a few scrambled thoughts had gone through her head: "I have to leave," "I won't be able to think of what to say to those geeky IT guys," "The woman sitting across from me will look great and monopolize the conversation," followed by "That's good as I won't have to talk" and "My hands will start to shake and I will make a mess of my food," followed by "At least I have on a dark-colored dress."

THOUGHTS, FEELINGS, AND ACTIONS RECORD

Situation (date, time, event)	Automatic thought(s)	Feelings (include intensity, rating from 0–100)	Actions/behaviors

It was also a bit tricky to determine her emotions since the panic she had felt upon arriving almost immediately subsided once she was in the washroom. She put down "panicky" 80/100, "awkward and embarrassed" 70/100, and "frozen" 75/100, and then returned to the thoughts column to add "My mind will go blank and I will stumble over my words." The actions/behaviors column was the easiest to complete as it was clear that she had headed for the washroom, and then into one of the stalls, avoiding interacting with anyone on the way there. After filling in her chart, her next action was to read through it and take some deep breaths to help calm herself down. She then realized she could request a change in the seating arrangements and immediately felt better.

Later in the evening Jody reviewed her self-monitoring chart and realized she had taken a very positive step in completing it—it helped her become more aware of her thoughts and feelings. She saw that her immediate tendency was to want to leave, which she had frequently done in the past. She also realized that while she felt nauseous, she had not vomited, which had also occurred in the past. Although going to the washroom was a temporary form of leaving, this short-term avoidant strategy proved to be very helpful as it provided her with personal space and privacy and the opportunity to sort through her reactions and reduce her panicky feelings by taking some slow, deep breaths.

You too will be able to separate your reactions into thoughts, feelings, and actions and clear up the blur when anxiety strikes. The self-monitoring process forces you to slow down and be more aware, which in and of itself is a useful strategy. You will then start to have specific ideas of what to do differently. But it's important to go through the entire process of looking at each component of your anxiety in the situation at hand. If Jody had simply thought "I'm feeling anxious at this party," leaving or trying to reduce her feelings of anxiety would have been her only choice. She could also have slowed down her thoughts with deep breathing to reduce her sense of panic, but she would not have figured out what to do to resolve the problem that led to the panic. As it happened, once Jody went through the self-monitoring process and her fear subsided, she sorted out some options to deal with the situation so she felt more comfortable during the evening. She ultimately chose to change her seat.

The key to successful self-monitoring (other than just doing it!) is to analyze specific situations. If you don't know the details of what is happening, it's not possible to change. Over time, you will likely start to see some patterns in your reactions. For example, Jody noticed right away that her anxiety was higher in the formal restaurant than it might have been at a casual self-serve buffet. She realized it was helpful to be able to choose where and with whom to sit. If she had either left right away or forced herself to "just get through it" and stay in her assigned seat, she might not have had these realizations. If she had left right away, her anxiety would have probably dropped due to the relief, but she might have felt guilty at leaving Emily behind and frustrated and disappointed with herself. If she had forced herself to remain at the first table where she was seated and was anxious throughout the evening, her negative thoughts about herself could have been reinforced ("I have nothing to say" or "I don't have anything in common with these people"). Once you understand your typical patterns, you're in a position to take charge. In the future, Jody is likely to be more proactive with seating arrangements, including asking a friend to help out. She can consider the type of restaurant, the people involved, and other factors that contribute to her anxiety.

> Knowledge is power and leads to improved coping.

But It All Happens So Fast!

It's common to struggle to be aware of automatic thoughts and feelings as well as to differentiate between them. As thoughts and feelings happen so quickly and almost at the same time, they are easy to miss. Separating them, however, empowers you. You'll be able to see that, even though the sequence may be the opposite, *typically a feeling is the result of a thought*. Here are some ways in which to sort out your thoughts and feelings and to figure out the difference between them.

What Are You Thinking?

Automatic thoughts are those fleeting verbal reactions in our minds that we have all the time without really noticing or thinking about them. They are our own personal narration of our experiences. They can be completely neutral and factual ("I see on my phone that it is 8:38 A.M."), positively tinged ("I really like the daily special that I saw posted in the cafeteria"), or negatively skewed ("They probably won't cook the special the way I like it"). Automatic thoughts can be about the situation itself, you, or other people. They can be both words or images and usually trigger other automatic thoughts, which trigger yet more thoughts. Memories may come to mind, such as thinking of a similar place, situation, or personal experience.

It can be tricky to figure out automatic thoughts, as they do happen so quickly. Automatic thoughts are not the same as underlying beliefs. For example, the automatic thought "I can't think of anything to say, and my mind is a blank" is probably related to a belief that it is important to talk to others and to make social connections in life. For the purposes of self-monitoring, don't worry about figuring out the underlying beliefs. Just try to catch some of the thoughts as they come into your mind.

What Are You Feeling?

Feelings come and go and affect us all the time. As noted earlier, they can be relatively stable or quite volatile. There is a broad range of human emotions, and they all occur on a continuum from mild to intense. Intense emotions can make it more difficult to think clearly. Our mind interprets how we feel and gives it a label. Some people are much more aware of their emotional state than others are—they could be said to have a larger emotional vocabulary. Some people prefer words to help identify emotions, and some prefer pictures such as emoticons.

How to Sort Out Your Thoughts and Feelings

Strategy 1: Check Out Pictures Representing Emotions

If you're not sure how you feel, try looking at the emojis on your cell phone. Emoticons or emojis are easy to use, and most people have access to them on their laptops or phones. Seeing the facial expressions in a comical way can help you identify the feelings expressed. Many emotion pictures and charts are available online. It can be helpful to have a fridge magnet or poster as a visual reminder.

Strategy 2: Increase Your Emotional Vocabulary

Many resources can help you identify feelings such as The Feelings Wheel (*Feelingswheel.com*), which helps put words to emotions and increase your emotional vocabulary. It's useful to have lots of options. Check out *psychpage.com/learning/library/assess/feelings.html* for ways to increase your emotion words.

Strategy 3: Say the Words Out Loud

Look at a list of emotions and try to say the words out loud. What do you feel at this moment? If you're in a private place, say it out loud several times, first in a whisper, then a bit louder and louder. There is an added benefit to verbalizing the words—naming emotions can actually help reduce them. Dr. Daniel Siegel, one of the first scientists to show support for this simple strategy, called it "name it to tame it." How do you feel after you have named the emotion and repeated it out loud? Is the emotion the same or different? Is it less intense or more intense?

Strategy 4: Practice

The next time someone asks you how you are, even in the grocery store, try to respond with a feeling word. "Okay" is not a feeling! "Tired," "happy," and "excited about the weekend" are possible options. Do this exercise for a full day—saying the words out loud helps awareness.

Strategy 5: Learn to Distinguish between Thoughts and Feelings

It's also quite normal for people to say "I feel . . ." and the feeling is actually a thought. The sentence "I feel that . . ." is usually a thought rather than a feeling, such as "I feel that I should not have come." Don't worry about getting it "right"—just get some thoughts and feelings down on a chart. It's much easier to figure it out once it's down in black and white.

Strategy 6: Be Curious

It can be interesting to practice awareness of feelings—ask yourself how you feel right now. It's quite common to have neutral or low intensities of emotion. That's probably the natural state of feeling! Some people have more up and down feelings, and others are more stable. Lots of times, when others ask "How are you doing?" you might respond with "okay" or "fine." Remember that these are not feelings.

Strategy 7: Try Body Sensations

If it's difficult for you to identify feelings, try body sensations such as an itch, warmth or cold, muscle tension, or a tickle in your throat. Body awareness can help get you started. What sensations do you have in this moment?

PRACTICE EXERCISE 1: Visualize being Jody

Imagine yourself in Jody's situation, walking through the door of the restaurant. Put yourself into the image as vividly as you can. What is the name of the restaurant? What is the décor like? What are you wearing? Do you notice any smells? Sounds? What is Emily saying? How do you feel? What is your first thought? Second thought? What do you see? Visualize the details of the scene before you imagine yourself heading off to the washroom. Picture yourself going into the washroom, feeling nauseous, and heading into the stall. Take a deep breath. Do you feel a bit better? Imagine yourself taking out your phone and pulling up a self-monitoring chart. Separate your reactions into thoughts, feelings, and actions. This brief exercise can help you figure out the difference between the thoughts and feelings that happen very quickly and automatically.

PRACTICE EXERCISE 2: Visualize your own example

Think of a situation that you find difficult and that leads to anxiety for you. Take a moment to think of something that happened in the past few days. Be as specific as possible—it could be meeting someone in person for the first time after you have talked on a dating app, or asking your boss for a promotion and a raise in pay, or running into a neighbor while out for a walk and not knowing what to say to them.

- Imagine yourself being back in this situation—let your imagination be as vivid as possible and put yourself into it fully. What happens? How does your body feel? What emotions do you experience? What are your thoughts? What do you do? What do you do next? How do you feel after your action? What are your next thoughts?
- How anxious do you feel in this situation? Rate your anxiety from 0 (complete calm) to 100 (worst anxiety I have ever felt) using the scale presented earlier in the chapter (page 34). Think of 20 as alert, 50 as moderate anxiety, and 70 as high anxiety. What other emotions do you have, and how intense are they?
- What thoughts and actions go along with these feelings? (See the cognitive behavioral triangle on page 32.) What do you do?
- Would you prefer to avoid any of these imagined actions?

   This exercise can help you sort out your reactions as well as determine what level of anxiety you can tolerate before being tempted to avoid situations. Some people avoid readily where others power through.

Self-Monitoring in Real Life—Making It Practical

Many of my clients have said that self-monitoring is helpful but not always convenient or practical. You cannot always stop what you're doing and pull out a self-monitoring form—also called a thought record—or use an app on your phone! There are, however, many ways to make self-monitoring work for you. Just make sure you include the "key ingredients"—the situation, your automatic thoughts, feelings, and actions.

Tip 1: Use Your Favorite Method

If you prefer paper, keep a small pad with you. Alternatively, you could set up a thought record on your phone or laptop. Some people use phone apps, such as MoodKit. Another idea could be to do a voice recording on your phone. Use whatever method or technology works best for you.

Tip 2: Keep It Simple

Many people customize their own records, but I would strongly advise you to keep it simple and straightforward. The more complicated the format, the less likely you are to complete it. I had a client create a very thorough, color-coded digital spreadsheet with drop-down options. While it was very thoughtful and creative, it was too complicated to use effectively for very long. I have had many clients create their own charts in a way that suits them.

Tip 3: Get It Out of Your Mind

You may think you will just remember what happened and be able to go through it in your mind later on. It is far better to write it down—seeing it "outside your mind" in black and white will help you be more objective and see things more clearly.

Tip 4: Keep It Private

Keeping your self-monitoring records private is important for many people. The use of your phone is very helpful in this regard—other people don't have access to it and you could use it for self-monitoring in a public space without anyone being the wiser. Self-monitoring looks much like any other activity, such as scrolling through social media and adding a few comments, so no one needs to know what you are doing!

Tip 5: Do It Quickly and Regularly

Complete the self-monitoring as soon as possible, as memory is fallible and biases may happen quickly. In this way, you can start to understand situations as they occur and see that there are other options in how you think and what you do. Most people do self-monitoring regularly when they start working on change and then are able to go through the steps quickly in their mind once it becomes routine.

Tip 6: Keep It Structured

Self-monitoring is not the same as journaling. Writing in a journal can mean many different things and can have numerous benefits, but typically it's far less structured and situation-specific than the type of monitoring discussed in this chapter. In my experience, people tend to write in journals when they are feeling sad or anxious. When reviewed afterward, journal entries can give a distorted perspective of situations as the notes are not kept in an organized or regular pattern. This can make it seem that life is actually worse than it is! Certainly, self-monitoring can be done in one of the lovely journals that are sold in bookstores. If that option appeals to you, go for it!

What You Can Learn by Comparing Predictions to Reality

When you're anxious about an upcoming event, you experience certain thoughts and feelings and can decide what you might do to manage the anxiety during the event. It's always important to look at the situation after the fact too, because you may very well have predicted very different results than what actually transpired. What happened when the actions you planned were taken? For people with anxiety many automatic thoughts are about the future, starting with "I will," "It might," or "Others will." Because these are future-oriented thoughts, and whatever they predict has not yet occurred, they are by definition untrue and untested. Try using the Thoughts, Feelings, and Actions

Record from this book to observe how different actual events can be from what you might predict.

PRACTICE EXERCISE 3: Predictions versus reality

Imagine that you're in your office about 15 minutes before a meeting. About 10 people will be in the conference room, including your boss, and you're going to present the results of a project that you've been working on for several months. While the project didn't turn out perfectly you are pleased with your work and the results, but you are worried that you won't be able to communicate very well. Here is an example of what you might enter into a thoughts, feelings, and actions record before the meeting begins. Notice that you're thinking about what might happen—how you may feel and what you could do to manage your anxiety. You are making a lot of predictions and entering the automatic thoughts in the record.

THOUGHTS, FEELINGS, AND ACTIONS RECORD (before meeting)

Situation (date, time, event)	Automatic thought(s)	Feelings (include intensity, rating from 0–100)	Actions/behaviors
Sitting in my office waiting for the 10:00 meeting. It is 9:45 A.M., March 14.	I won't be able to express myself very well. There will be challenging questions from my boss. I will stumble over my words and won't be able to think of what to say. Others will laugh at me. I will get fired for making too many mistakes and not being able to present my work. I will run out of the meeting.	Nervous—75 Apprehensive—80 Anticipation—40 Terrified—85 Embarrassed—60 Worried—65	Practice the first few sentences of the talk. Go over the PowerPoint slides. Poke my head into my next-door neighbor's office and walk to the meeting with her. Think of ways to respond to predictable questions. Realize that it's okay to say "I don't know." Take my water bottle to the meeting in case I get a dry mouth.

Here's an example of what you might record about your thoughts, feelings, and actions after the meeting regarding what actually happened.

THOUGHTS, FEELINGS, AND ACTIONS RECORD (after meeting)

Situation (date, time, event)	Automatic thought(s)	Feelings (include intensity, rating from 0–100)	Actions/behaviors
In my office, 11:15 A.M., March 14.	Well, I'm glad that's over! I didn't do a great job, but at least I got through it. No one laughed (out loud anyway!). I was able to respond to some of the questions. When I said "I don't know" to one question, another person had the answer. My boss smiled at me at the end of the meeting, so perhaps I won't be fired (today anyway!).	Relief—90 Embarrassed—50 Nervous—40 Tired—60 Proud—30	Close my eyes and take a breather. Post my slides on the shared drive so that others can review them. Send a message letting my colleagues know that I've posted the slides. Ask my colleague next door what she thought of my presentation. Think of a possible rewarding activity for the evening.

In the post-meeting exercise example, you can see that most of the thoughts are no longer future oriented. Some of the feelings are the same, but their intensity is reduced. The nervous or embarrassed feelings are still about the future ("I won't be fired today" implies that it could still happen in the near future). A key point is that anxiety is a future-oriented emotion, tending to escalate just before and at the beginning of a feared situation, that can easily lead to avoidance ("I'm so terrified that I can't manage it, so I'll just not go"). Anxious thoughts are predictions about the future and not focused on the present. Just as in the examples above, it can be helpful to compare a thoughts, feelings, and actions record from before an event to a record completed after the event occurred. This exercise can help you see that your predictions are not the same as reality!

Early in my career I heard an expert say that anxiety is about the future and depression is about the past. That statement rang true then and has stuck with me. While this book is not focused on depression, many socially anxious people have regrets about opportunities not taken and sadness about events in the past.

The Value of an Outsider's Perspective

Sometimes it's hard to figure it all out—what thoughts, feelings, and actions are involved in your social anxiety and how your predictions differ from what actually unfolds. It can help to get someone else's thoughts. While no one else knows what you think or how you feel, they can comment on your actions and provide their view on your strengths and how you counteract your anxiety. Others' opinions may be quite different from yours and provide good information. As in the office example in the preceding exercise, you may know someone whose opinion you trust and who was present at the event that caused you anxiety, and you could ask them what they thought. You may have noticed all of your mistakes while others didn't even see or hear them. Take their opinion as a piece of information. If you talk to someone who wasn't present, try to provide an unbiased description of what happened. It can take courage to talk to someone else about a situation that led to anxiety, but it's extremely useful to get multiple perspectives.

Consider the Situation: Context Matters

Situations do not occur in a vacuum, and the context makes a huge difference to how your social anxiety comes into play. Most people know this intuitively, but it will become much more evident when you start self-monitoring. Here are some of the considerations to think about.

What Is at Stake?

If you give a presentation for a job interview, the stakes are high and most people would be nervous. If you are showing a slideshow of your vacation photos to friends, the stakes are not very high, but it's easy to have negative thoughts. These thoughts could include that your pictures are not very good or that the vacation was not that interesting and your friends may judge your choices or photography skills. If the situation is your attending a lecture where you are not expected to participate, the stakes are low and you're not likely to feel very anxious. The stakes go up, though, and anxiety may start to creep higher if you decide to ask a question or you're interested in talking to someone else who's there. If the situation involves taking a long hike in the mountains when no one is around, a socially anxious person is not likely to feel uncomfortable, whereas a person who believes there may be hidden dangers (for example, bears) or is worried about their fitness may be terrified. As you are aware, people who struggle with social anxiety fear judgment, so the social context is very important.

Who Are You With?

Situations may involve other people with whom you share a history. Sharing a history may make your preferred response to a given situation either easier or much more difficult, depending on the relationship you have with the person. For example, if your relationship with the other person is positive and you think they are likely to be supportive, you'll often find it easier to take risks. At times this shared history can complicate your reactions, however, because thinking you know how the other person will respond may get factored into your predictions. And those predictions could turn out to be accurate or inaccurate! You can even make predictions about people you've never met before, because it's human nature to make assumptions based on first impressions, visual cues, or the location you're in. Jody, for example, made assumptions about the two men who worked in IT based on minimal information. You may find yourself gravitating toward or away from an interaction based on your assumptions. Just as your read of people that you know well can be inaccurate, your first impressions of strangers may be wrong. Be open to the possibility that you don't always know what others are like!

Consider how you feel and what thoughts you have when you're with the people you typically see during the day. People you've never met may be easier to approach as you may have fewer expectations and assumptions about how the interaction will proceed. These expectations will, of course, depend on many factors, such as where the interactions occur. I have had clients tell me they feel much less anxious traveling far from home, even in a different country, where no one knows them and they are not expected to talk. They reported that it was "freeing" and allowed them to be more rather than less sociable. People may feel more comfortable in a waiting room at a mental health clinic as they know that everyone who is waiting also has mental health struggles. Or they may feel less comfortable as they are worried that someone may recognize them and make judgments.

What Is the Setting?

There are lots of other patterns that you can see from your self-observations, and these can help you understand the components of your responses to social anxiety. Like Jody, many anxious people feel more comfortable in casual social situations, often when they are outdoors where there is a lot of space to move around. That way, there are choices of where to go and who to talk to or places to escape to and be less visible. On the other hand, many anxious people dislike "cocktail party chatter" or what is commonly called *networking* as the conversations are unstructured and it is not clear what to talk about. Structured interactions tend to be easier as in these situations it is clearer what is expected of you.

PRACTICE EXERCISE 4: Rank situations from most to least comfortable

This exercise helps you understand some of your reactions and realize that they are on a continuum from least to most difficult. Almost all reactions are like this, and figuring it out will give you a "way in" to making the situation a bit easier for yourself. You may also see that there are already situations that you can handle with a moderate degree of comfort.

List some sample situations that you would put in the following categories, from most to least comfortable:

Most comfortable:

Moderately comfortable:

Moderately uncomfortable:

Most uncomfortable:

Ryan preferred to go for long walks late at night so that he would not run into people and be expected to talk. He felt most comfortable interacting with peers in the context of gaming as it was clear what the topic of the chats would be. He felt moderately comfortable talking to his mother and slightly less comfortable talking to his father. Lisa felt comfortable at work at the shopping center when very few people were around. When she noticed teenagers out shopping in groups, she tended to avoid looking at them as she thought that they would judge her. She felt more comfortable walking the periphery of the parking lot and enjoyed interacting with young families with children.

PRACTICE EXERCISE 5: Notice how the situation affects you

Imagine that you are riding on a city transit bus. You have a seat, but the bus is full and lots of people are standing up. You are looking down, minding your own business, but feel self-conscious and wonder if you should give up your seat. As you look at the floor, it feels as though many eyes are staring at you and people are wondering why you don't stand up and offer your seat to someone else. You feel guilty and start to shift your position to look out the window. Force yourself to lift your eyes and look around. Notice who is nearby. How many people are staring at you? What is the expression on their faces? Are they looking at anyone else? How many people are looking out the window? Talking to someone else? On their phones? Is there a good reason here to feel guilty? Do you feel more self-conscious when looking down or looking up?

This exercise helps you understand the importance of the social environment around you and how your behavior affects how you feel. Most people feel much more uncomfortable and anxious when avoiding contact with others. Self-monitoring can encourage you to look around, and doing so can reveal a great deal. You are likely to notice that other people are not looking at you or even noticing much other than what is in their immediate vicinity (especially their screens!).

Consider Personal Characteristics: You Matter

Everyone lives in different circumstances. We all have unique barriers that get in the way and qualities that can help us move ahead in living our best lives. Some people have more privileges than others, including adequate financial support and safe housing, good health, and being part of a majority group. Others contend with obstacles that make change more challenging. It is certainly hard to focus on dealing with social anxiety if you do not have money to buy medicine, food, or safe housing. On the other hand, necessity may force some people to do things they would prefer to avoid, and this may turn out to be a good thing.

Earlier in this chapter, we looked at how negative thoughts and predictions can be identified through self-monitoring. These negative thoughts can be accurate. A thought that others are looking at you and judging you negatively can be accurate. The thought that others may not like you could be true. People can judge and have negative thoughts about themselves as well as about others.

Life is not the same for everyone, and it is certainly not fair. Most people who are part of a visible minority group have likely experienced discrimination and intolerance from other people. If you have mobility issues and use a wheelchair, life is going to be more complicated, and you face physical barriers to getting around. Many people live with histories of trauma, societal injustice, and economic disparity. Any or all of these obstacles can make change more challenging and have to be considered in working to live your best life. While some obstacles can be overcome, some have to be accepted and some may be best dealt with on a societal level through social justice initiatives.

We all have characteristics that can help as well as those that get in the way. Determination, wanting wholeheartedly to live your best life, and tenacity are all important characteristics. Curiosity about yourself, other people, and the world around you is helpful. The desire to learn can help you try new activities and talk to different people. The realization that other people struggle and have their own fears can be eye-opening and help you feel less alone. The ability to not only tolerate but welcome surprises is helpful, especially as life truly is unpredictable. The only certainty is uncertainty. That statement can be exhilarating and terrifying at the same time!

For more self-awareness, ask yourself the following questions:

- What are the major obstacles that you face in your life at present?
- What are some ways that they could be either overcome or reduced?
- If they are unchangeable, can you imagine yourself accepting them?
- What are five personal characteristics that you have that are helpful?
- If you have trouble identifying your helpful characteristics, can you think of someone that you could ask this question of? Even if you are able to answer the question, getting someone else's perspective can be illuminating.
- Think of ways in which these qualities might help you make changes. For example, tenacity is a real asset and can be manifested as persistence!

Moving Forward

In this chapter we have discussed the details of understanding yourself, your life situation, and things that might either get in the way or help you along the way. Through self-monitoring, you will be able to separate your thoughts, feelings, and actions and work toward shifting them in more positive directions. Practice labeling your feelings through the use of emoticons or words, whichever you prefer. Say the emotion words out loud when you are by yourself. Slow down and create space between the immediate reaction and what happens next. It's an important first step to slow down enough that you can reduce some of the initial first reactions. Once you do that, you can figure out the next steps. Keeping track for yourself or getting other opinions helps you get a different perspective on what's happening. Now that you have a deeper understanding, the next chapter will turn to how to set goals that work and keep you on track toward living your best life.

3

gearing up for change— and making it stick

You have now identified the ways in which social anxiety is limiting your life and want to reduce its hold on you by making positive changes. You have learned that social anxiety is not mysterious or uncontrollable. Your self-monitoring has shown that there are clear patterns to the problems that can be interrupted. You are gearing up for change!

We all change in response to our environment and through influences such as the media, the culture that surrounds us, and our relationships. We often don't recognize these changes as they can be subtle and happen gradually. You probably have heard the saying "change is the only constant," which is borne out over and over. Change happens all the time and in different ways. At times, fears reduce or go away completely without your even noticing. Childhood fears, including social anxiety, may decrease with exposure and experience. At the same time, fears can develop and increase, and it's important to be in control and aware of these responses.

Social anxiety in adults usually does not improve on its own without effort. The key to helping yourself is to be purposeful and planful about change. Many people say "I want to feel better" or "I want to be less anxious" but are not sure how to achieve that outcome. Because that is what feeling better is—an outcome of some type of action or change in thoughts. It is difficult to think of how to get to that end point. A person must do something or think differently to feel better. Just as taking an antibiotic reduces symptoms of an infection with the outcome of feeling better, taking action to counteract social anxiety generally leads to improved functioning and lower anxiety over time.

This chapter will discuss change, some possible targets for change, and how to set goals that are within your control. Deliberate change happens through working on the day-to-day details of life. Small steps toward change practiced frequently and over time lead to lasting improvement.

Now that you understand social anxiety and have learned about your patterns through self-monitoring, you are ready to set goals that are important to you and consistent with your values. Setting goals and following through with them puts you in the driver's seat.

> Be deliberate and planful about change.
> The outcome is feeling better.

> Work toward the change you want
> with effective strategies.

Know What Changes Are Most Important to You

It takes effort and persistence to work toward goals, so it's very important to think about the reasons to overcome your fears. Why are you interested in change? What is most important to you? No doubt you want to feel better, but let's think about what else you will gain. Do you want to return to school, apply for a job, improve your social life, or generally feel more at ease in the world? You're not likely to be able to feel better without making some changes in your life.

Consistent steps toward change take ongoing work, which requires maintaining motivation. Most of us have set goals to start something on a Monday and then lost momentum a few days later. It is important to keep in mind the big picture and the reasons why you want to make changes. Your goals and the values that guide your life should be consistent with each other. If someone or something else—like a family member, a therapist, a job—is guiding change, your efforts probably won't be successful. To be reachable, goals should be not only attainable but also consistent with what you want in your life and aligned with your values. They should come from you.

Be Brave—Change Requires Risk

Most people with social anxiety place a high value on connections with others, and you may feel robbed of the relationships that you both crave and fear. Developing social connections takes courage and skills and involves uncertain outcomes. New relationships begin tentatively and develop gradually. The rewards for sticking it out include increased confidence and the satisfaction of making the effort and taking the risks.

Please remember that most people struggle with close connections. Sharing hopes, dreams, and emotions with others can lead to feelings of vulnerability. It's easy to have fears of judgment or rejection. Socially anxious people tend to have more difficulty with starting new relationships and navigating the beginning of them but tend to be loyal friends or employees once in relationships. I have had clients tell me that if they could just magically skip over the early parts of initiating connections, they would be just fine!

Even though you know the outcome of a richer life is probably worth the trouble, it's scary and difficult to know how to get there. You have already learned how tempting avoidance is when the short-term relief it provides seems far preferable to the day-to-day challenge of the hard work of change. This is why it's important to know what's most important to you and have a clear plan: Being able to keep your values and plan in mind while working toward change can counteract any feelings of vulnerability and risk that arise. Sometimes where you are seems like the beginning of a story and where you want to be is the conclusion, but it's difficult to figure out how to get to that end point. Setting goals that are aligned with your values is like figuring out the plotline of your life.

Know Your Values

When setting important goals, it's a good idea to back up and think about your values first. It doesn't make sense to work hard to make changes without figuring out what's most important to you. Then your overall life goals can be based on your values, and the goals can be translated into specifics in your day-to-day life to fill in a roadmap for change.

Values are what you strive to live for and give meaning to your life. Living in ways that are closely aligned with your values is being true to yourself. This is sometimes called *living with integrity*. Values provide guidance for decision making and actions.

Some commonly held values are those related to social connections, achievement, creativity, spirituality, and independence. Health, curiosity, and integrity are other values. Several tools are available to help you identify your values. For a free online values assessment, try Personal Values (*https://personalvalu.es*). What are the most important values for you? If you had to choose between learning, independence, compassion for others, pleasure and enjoyment, success, power and recognition, safety and security, accountability, and friends, family, and belonging, what would your top three choices be?

Translate Values into Goals

Values should guide your overall goals. If someone else suggests that you work on relationships but relationships are not that important to you, you will not work very hard at making friends. Being creative or being competent in your work may be more aligned with your values. Achievement and success are crucial to some people, but not at all to others.

Overall goals are often abstract or vague—"I want to improve my social life to make new friends." These broad goals are fine to start with, as long as you make them concrete so you can work on them day to day. Narrowing a broad, abstract goal to something more specific and concrete—"I will attend the party on Friday night for two hours"—allows you to make measurable steps toward your values-based goals. See the examples in the chart on page 58.

VALUES VERSUS GOALS

	Descriptions	Example(s)
Values	• Are pursued for their own sake • Are never permanently realized • Cannot be evaluated or judged • Must be chosen	1. Being a good friend 2. Being physically healthy 3. Being courageous
Abstract Goals	• Work in the service of values • Are often broadly applicable • Do not refer to one specific type of behavior	1. Supporting and being more connected to my friend(s) 2. Exercising regularly 3. Doing things that make me anxious or frightened
Concrete Goals	• Are concrete behaviors that work in the service of an abstract goal	1. Phoning my friend Dawn, who is depressed, once a week to ask how she is doing 2. Getting up at 7 A.M. on Monday and Wednesday to go work on the elliptical trainer at the gym for 30 minutes 3. Greeting the cashier at the grocery store and asking her three questions once a week

Unpublished chart developed by Caelin White, PhD, and used with permission.

Move from the Abstract to the Concrete

To set goals for change, it's important to narrow the focus from the general to the specific details of your life that are affected by social anxiety. You've learned through self-monitoring what these details are, and you can use them to guide your concrete goals. These concrete goals can then be made into daily steps.

Small, frequent steps are easier to take than occasional big steps and feel less overwhelming. They are also far more effective over the long term. Just imagine for a moment that you were afraid of public speaking and only had opportunities to speak in public once every year or two. It could take a long time to rack up enough experience to reduce your fear. Another option would be to figure out ways to incorporate speaking up into daily life. So how do you integrate practice into daily life to achieve your goals? It takes planning.

Make a Plan: Consulting the Cognitive Behavioral Triangle

Let's start by looking at which parts of the cognitive behavioral triangle in Chapter 2 you want to target for change: feelings, thoughts, or actions? How you feel physically and emotionally affects how you think and what actions or inactions you choose to take. The goal of change in your daily life can be to change feelings, thoughts, or actions, the situation itself, or some combination. Typically, goals work on shifting thoughts and actions in order to shift feelings. You may decide, for example, to change your actions so that you don't fear certain types of social situations as intensely as you do now. Or you may work on challenging your negative thoughts about yourself to be more comfortable with others.

Lisa wanted to feel more comfortable at work and improve her relationships with her colleagues. She set a concrete goal of changing her actions by initiating contact with coworkers every day. She first noticed that her colleague Jon seemed to ignore her, which made her anxious, but she persisted and ended up realizing that his response was not within her control. She tried to be observant and continue her self-monitoring. After a week or two, she felt less anxiety and a greater ability to observe others due to being less distracted by her own anxious reactions. She noticed that Jon tended to be distractible, and became less likely to take his responses to her personally.

Did Lisa feel more comfortable at work and have better relationships with her colleagues right away? No. But her persistence was building small changes that could eventually help her reach those goals. The key is to set goals that work.

Help Yourself Change: Set Goals That Work

Have you ever set a goal that you didn't achieve? Almost everyone has set unrealistic or unattainable goals—think of resolutions for the New Year. Many people set resolutions such as changing jobs, improving their social life, or eating more healthy foods. These resolutions are quite broad and somewhat abstract. They may be completely aligned with your values. But what does it mean to improve your social life? What foods are healthy versus unhealthy? Change-related goals need to be defined. Many people lose their motivation and incentive for change by the end of January, often because their goals weren't specific enough to be attainable.

Make Goals Concrete by Targeting Behavior

Personal change is difficult to achieve and especially to sustain over the long term unless it focuses on behavior change. Health improvements can come from behavioral shifts like changing your diet. An improved social life can come from behavior changes like sitting at a table with other people at work and starting a conversation. Your own behavior is within your control. As Lisa discovered, she could experience some changes in her comfort level at work by repeatedly initiating contact with colleagues, but she couldn't reduce her anxiety directly by controlling how they responded to her. Feelings are difficult to change directly, but you can work toward changes in anxiety through changes in your behavior. While you can influence others by how you act, you cannot change or control their responses.

Set Goals That Take the Situation into Account

As noted above, you can not only target the three parts of the cognitive behavioral triangle to effect change but also become aware of and consider the situation. Situations have a big influence on our behaviors.

Ryan didn't like his parents nagging him to move ahead in his life and look for a job, although he grudgingly agreed with them. He secretly admired his parents, who had worked hard and achieved financial security, and decided that he valued independence and achievement. He wasn't sure how to go about attaining those things but decided he should act. Ryan chose getting a job as his overall goal, and set an initial concrete goal of taking an online tutorial on how to write a résumé (week 1) and then spending 15 minutes a day working on his résumé (week 2). He then set another goal of making a list of 10 possible places to apply for a service-related job (week 3), sending out 10 résumés (week 4), and following up with each potential employer a week later. All of these steps were within his control and could lead to obtaining a job.

To reach the goal of getting a job, Ryan had to work backwards and consider all of the steps toward that end point. It would have been easy to become discouraged and lose momentum, but if he had success with the first goal, he would be more likely to work on the second one. Picking attainable steps made him feel like he was making progress.

Use SMART Goals to Achieve Success

Therapists sometimes use the acronym SMART as a reminder for helpful goal setting. Ideally goals would be **Specific, Measurable, Achievable, Relevant,** and **Realistic** and have a clear **Time frame.** It is important to know exactly what is to be done—for example, "I will say hello to three people at work this morning" versus "I will try to be friendly." The goal to greet three others this morning is likely to be SMART as it is specific, can be counted, and has a clear time frame. It is probably achievable unless no other people are present to be greeted. It is relevant only if it's something you want to work on and is important to you.

Consider changes for yourself. An overall goal is some realistic change that is achievable within a specific time period. The time frame is very important as it is common to put things off, thinking that there is plenty of time in the future to work toward the goal. SMART goals work well because they can be broken down into specific steps, they are within your control, and it is clear to you when and if the goal is reached. Specific goals are steps toward an overall goal and may include the ways in which the overall goal is to be achieved.

PRACTICE EXERCISE 1: Turning your overall goal into a SMART goal

You can use these steps to make sure any of your goals regarding reducing social anxiety are SMART. Try it with an overall goal right now. Think of a social goal that you have been considering, such as making new friends at school.

Step 1. Ask yourself these questions about your goal:
S = Is it Specific?
M = Is it Measurable?
A =Is it Achievable?
R = Is it Relevant to you and Realistic?
T = What is the Time Frame?

Step 2. State your overall goal and then recast it as specific concrete goals.

Overall Goal: _____

_____

Specific Concrete Goals: _____

_____

Build the Skills You Need to Reach Your Goals

Once you have some ideas about your overall and specific goals, ask yourself if you need any skills to achieve them. Do you struggle with certain types of social skills, setting boundaries for yourself, or frequent negative thoughts about other people? You may need to learn specific skills so that you can make the changes you want. There is no doubt at all that lots of practice will be required to develop proficiency, and proficiency builds confidence. That is true for all of us.

Think of a fear that you had in the past that you no longer have—examples could be driving a car, riding a bicycle, or skiing down a mountain. These are all things that people may fear if they haven't experienced them or don't have the required skills. Learning skills and practicing them repeatedly leads to increased confidence. These changes reduce fear. Fear makes sense if a situation carries risks. Hurtling down a mountain on skis is risky without skills (and good equipment!). Perceived risks lead to fear, and these risks can be physical, emotional, psychological, or social.

While it's easier to consider physical risks, social situations also entail risks, such as the possibility of unpredictable responses to our actions, and require many different types of skills. It's more difficult to predict how people will respond than inanimate objects! Social risks involve other people, who can be unpredictable and hard to read.

Adrian, a college student, wants to ask Lin to share notes and study for an upcoming exam. If he predicts that she will say no and he will feel devastated, he is not going to ask. If he thinks there is a possibility she might say yes, and that he would be able to manage either way, he is going to try. If he has other options for people to study with, he will be less anxious. If he predicts that Lin will enthusiastically say yes, he will go for it!

Adrian might have the courage to ask Lin to study with him if he felt he had social skills to make his invitation appealing, as well as coping skills if she wasn't interested.

Taking social risks can be as simple as saying hello to a new person, asking someone out on a date, or initiating a friendship. It can be moving, changing schools, or deciding where to buy takeout food. People who are socially anxious fear social risk more than other types of risks. I knew someone who was able to skydive out of an airplane but not ask a person on a date. He was confident in his physical abilities but not his social ones. Socially anxious people may have thoughts that they will be perceived as needy and will be rejected and judged. To ask someone on a date certainly can lead to rejection, and it's safer (and lonelier) not to make that effort. All of these situations require skill as well as courage.

People tend to feel anxious if the estimated risk from doing something is greater than their presumed ability to cope with it. If you think your coping skills are low and the risk is high, it's going to be difficult to convince yourself to try! Anxious people tend to doubt their coping skills and overestimate the risks. (They also overestimate others' ability to cope, relative to their own.) Building skills through practice is very helpful.

Just like learning to drive, learning any skills including how to develop and navigate relationships takes time and practice. If you have ever studied a second language, especially as an adult, think about how much time and effort it took. Many people feel self-conscious and embarrassed when speaking a new language for fear of making mistakes or not being understood. But without repeated practice, it's impossible to acquire a language. It takes a great deal of practice to become proficient. People don't expect themselves to become fluent quickly without immersion in a language and culture. Remember this analogy when thinking about the development of skills to achieve social anxiety goals.

There are many types of skills that will help you achieve your goals. Later chapters in this book focus on skills to increase your exposure, challenge your thoughts, manage your physical responses, and improve your communication with others. Once you figure out your goals and the necessary skills, working on them step by step through practice builds confidence.

Taking Steps to Set Yourself Up for Success

As you start working on your goals and skills, you might find it helpful to use the following roadmap:

1. *Set an initial specific, concrete goal that is straightforward and attainable to provide motivation.* Examples include getting information online for a class that you are interested in signing up for, or texting someone who you feel comfortable with and proposing going for a walk on the weekend. Once you've taken a step, it's easier to continue. Small successes will make you feel good.

2. *Think of a goal that you have already met (it doesn't have to be regarding anxiety).* How did you do it? What worked? What got in the way? Write down the answers to these questions and think about what you might take from them to apply to social anxiety.

3. *Set a goal that you could work on right now and "just do it."* For example, turn around, smile, and say hello to a person sitting near you or send a quick text to a family member. Notice your reaction to this task.

4. *Take small steps every day.* They will become habitual over time, although we often underestimate how long habits take to form—at least a month or even more. If you find this fact frustrating, think of how long it took to develop social anxiety! Small daily steps add up to big steps.

5. *Keep track of these steps*—write them down, set up a folder on your phone, put check marks on the calendar. People who lack self-confidence often minimize their progress, and keeping track helps collect solid evidence to counteract this tendency.

6. *Keep track of your progress.* If you've kept track of your steps, it's easier to see how you're doing overall. Slow, gradual progress can be more difficult to notice than the bigger steps. Some people find it helpful to pick a regular time each week to assess how they've done over the previous week and then to think about plans for the upcoming week. Sunday evening is often a good time to do this planning.

7. *Reward yourself for your efforts rather than the outcome.* While the outcome is beyond your control, your efforts are not. If you tried something related to your goals, give yourself a pat on the back and lots of credit. Keep track of your efforts—they are what count.

8. *Don't beat yourself up if you did not try something one day or bowed out at the last minute.* It can be easy to give up if you've had a bad day, and it's important to see it as just one day (or even part of one day).

9. *Remember that no one is perfect when practicing new skills.* Give yourself permission to make mistakes and value imperfection. Learning cannot occur without it—be perfectly imperfect!

Notice How Your Behavior Responds to Your Environment

We change in ways that we do not necessarily plan or think about. Consider a time when you changed in response to your environment—these changes happen often without our really noticing. I can think of many examples from my own life. For instance, at one point I realized that I was drinking far too much coffee at work. A new machine had been installed very close to my office, and I walked by it several times a day, so it was very easy to be reminded of my caffeine affinity and to grab another cup. In addition, it was free! After I became aware of the change, it took a deliberate effort to reduce my consumption; sometimes I had to force myself to walk the other way so I would not pass the machine. We tend to gravitate toward things that are accessible, convenient, and easy. The sneaky part was that I hadn't even really noticed the change.

Observing how you react to your environment can help you take advantage of opportunities to use practical social skills that you haven't recognized need honing. We interact the most with people who are physically close to us and whom we see on a regular basis. If something is not in our immediate environment, we are far less likely to think of it. We have limited opportunities to engage in natural interactions if we are not around people very often, as happened during the COVID-19 pandemic and still happens as people continue to work from home. In-person interactions take deliberate effort and are easy to avoid as we tend to do what is convenient and easy. Many people have purchased a discounted membership at a gym that is inexpensive but inconveniently located, only to learn that they are not likely to go for a workout very often if it entails a drive or has limited hours or classes.

The interactions that we might have during a trip to the grocery store or coffee shop or merely walking down the street influence our mental health and provide opportunities for casual engagement with others. We communicate with others in many ways in addition to talking—through our facial expressions and body language as well as simply by being in the same place. All of these interactions make a difference in terms of our mental health and development and maintenance of interpersonal skills.

An important strategy is to set up your environment for success. Goals related to social anxiety require a person to have opportunities to interact with people. If you are seldom around people, it will be much more difficult. What can you do to make change more convenient?

> Our behaviors change in response
> to our daily environment.

Notice How Your Thoughts and Opinions Respond to Your Environment

Just as our behaviors change in response to our daily environment, so do our thoughts and opinions. If we are around people who express fearful thoughts, those comments have an influence on us and often increase our wariness. If we interact with people who have attitudes like ours, our attitudes are strengthened. Socially anxious people tend to believe that others judge them, which is easily reinforced either by other people or by the media. News stories often lead with sensational and negative headlines. Social media feeds are created by algorithms that provide information that is similar to what we already think. Our attitudes are shaped by our families, our friends, and the community and culture that surrounds us (both online and "in real life"). With limited opportunities to be around others of different opinions and backgrounds, a socially anxious person may struggle to see their thoughts as "just their opinion" and instead view them as fact. But thoughts are not facts. If these thoughts don't get challenged or tested, they will not be disconfirmed.

For example, if Jody, in her new position, keeps to herself at work and has thoughts that others don't like her, she will not have opportunities to find out otherwise. Her feelings of self-consciousness and thoughts that others are looking at her in negative ways will feel accurate even if no one is noticing her at all. It can be both a shock and a relief to realize how little other people notice as they are absorbed in their own worlds. Becoming aware of others' lack of attention can be quite liberating and help you overcome fears of change.

An important strategy that will be discussed in detail in Chapter 5 is to learn to be aware of your thoughts and to be open to the reality that "thoughts are not facts."

> **Our thoughts change in response to our daily environment.**

Take Gradual Steps toward Change

Jorge's overall goal was to be more at ease in group settings and not be held back by fears of judgment. He set a more specific goal of agreeing to public speaking opportunities. Jorge agreed to give the toast at an upcoming family wedding but had a difficult time thinking about how to help himself with this daunting task. While he had attended weddings and listened to toasts, he had never given one. He saw the people who gave these toasts as talented and articulate. He did work in an office environment with numerous other people and had a number of friends that he saw regularly. Consequently, there were opportunities to take if he chose to do so. Through conversations with a trusted and sensible friend, he came up with the following steps to take over the coming weeks:

1. *Do some research on what to include in a toast at a wedding—look up appropriate jokes, sayings, and quotes on the internet.*
2. *Look through old family photos and talk to his brothers to stimulate memories and stories.*
3. *Create an ideas folder on his laptop.*
4. *Ask a question or make a comment at all work meetings attended over the next month.*
5. *Offer to chair an upcoming meeting of a community nonprofit group that he belongs to.*
6. *Draft a two-minute speech on an interest that he has and practice it when alone sitting in the car (not driving).*
7. *Practice giving this speech to a trusted friend.*
8. *Practice giving this speech a second time and ask for feedback.*
9. *Practice giving this speech to a small group of people at a family dinner.*
10. *Practice several more times.*

Jorge created sensible steps that were attainable, within his control, and relevant to his overall plan of giving the speech. He worked to make them specific and set a time frame with reminders on his cell phone. The steps were likely to help increase his confidence.

Public speaking is not something most people do very often. Fears of low-frequency events are more difficult to overcome because regular practice can be hard to obtain. Situations such as fears of flying, poisonous snakes, elevators, or public speaking may not become relevant until you're expected to encounter these fears or the environment changes. A fear of flying does not interfere with your life unless you want to travel or are expected to do so for work or family events. It is easy to avoid elevators if you live on the main floor of a building and do not work in a high-rise. It would be a problem, however, if you did not apply for a good job because of the floor on which it was located.

Similarly, public speaking is less important if you work from home. There are lots of subtle ways, however, that fear of public speaking can interfere with your life, and Jorge gradually became aware of that as he began to work on his fear. He noticed, for example, that he avoided asking questions at meetings and was much more likely to send them to his supervisor by email. He hesitated to volunteer to be in leadership roles as that put him in the spotlight, and he avoided telling jokes even though he had a very good sense of humor. These issues were all related to his fear of public speaking although he had not thought of them in the same way.

Maintain Motivation for Change

TAKE SMALL STEPS

Most of us have started a project and let it go after a few days or weeks. It helps if there is a natural deadline, such as the wedding that Jorge was going to attend to give his toast, but otherwise it can be challenging to keep up the momentum for change. Maintaining motivation over time is crucial, and strategies to take small gradual steps over a long time are recommended rather than occasional big steps.

> Small successes increase motivation.

KEEP RECORDS

While self-monitoring over time helps you understand yourself, it is also important to keep records of what you do to reduce social anxiety. Consider starting a folder on your laptop or phone or putting together a physical folder or binder to put your records in. Even simple steps such as putting check marks on your calendar or keeping a phone counter (such as a Counter app) helps. Check marks on a calendar could indicate days when you tried something new, and a clicker could be a count of similar kinds of behavior.

> Setting up reminders that pop up each day
> is a good way to maintain momentum and motivation.

TAKE PRIDE IN YOUR WORK

To keep yourself moving forward, think about what you will gain by making changes for yourself. Not only will your life improve, but you will feel proud of yourself. Think of something that you have done in the past that was difficult to accomplish and that you now acknowledge and feel proud of. It might have been a trip that you took on your own, a course that you completed, or a new business relationship with a person you approached for help. It might have been picking up this book and learning more about yourself. There are pros and cons to any change, but living well is a definite advantage!

> Take pride in every effort that you make toward change.

VALUE YOURSELF AS YOU WORK ON CHANGE

It's important to accept and value who you are as a person while promoting change. You are worthy of change and worthy of living your best life. You have already made many changes in your life whether planned or unplanned.

> You are worth it.

DON'T PUT THINGS OFF

When you work on your goals, keep the present in mind and don't put things off. What can you do today to work toward a goal? What can you do right now? Sometimes we are surprised by what happens. These surprises can be good ones or not so good—it is important to be open to the possibilities. If life were totally predictable, it would be boring! Be open to surprises!

> Just do it!

USE THE "FOUR P'S" FORMULA

This formula is easy to remember and could be recorded somewhere on your phone. It is:

Patience + Persistence + Pacing = Progress

Taking small steps frequently (pacing), being patient and kind with yourself, and persisting across time are all helpful. *Pacing* is important, as many people tend to try to take big steps infrequently rather than small steps regularly. Imagine for a moment that you signed up to run a marathon. It would be sensible to develop a schedule and become more fit slowly and gradually. If you tried to run even half a marathon the first time you went out to exercise, you likely would be so tired and sore that you might give up! A goal of saying hello to three people every day becomes easier over time. To pace yourself in this way is doable and does not set you up for failure unless you do not encounter at least three people in an average day. If that is the case, set a different goal. On the other hand, a goal such as "have a meaningful conversation with a friend" is not only vague but is also an activity that cannot be done frequently.

Ensure that goals are begun from where you are now, rather than where you would like to be. Reward your efforts even if they do not work out perfectly. It is important to accept where you are right at this moment and to acknowledge both the efforts you make and the obstacles you encounter. Be *patient* and supportive of yourself while you try to be brave and work to provide opportunities for yourself to try new ways of being. In my opinion, *persistence* may be the most important part of the equation. Don't give up! If something doesn't work the first time, scale it back, try it again, or modify it. People who persist generally have good results. All of these qualities lead to *progress*.

Moving Forward

Now that you have learned about your own social anxiety and tried out self-monitoring in specific situations, setting goals, and maintaining your motivation for change, you are ready to move to learning strategies to deal with your emotional reactions, thoughts, and actions. These daily life strategies will help you achieve your goals and live your best life.

PART TWO

daily-life strategies for change in social anxiety

4

how to respond planfully to your feelings

Jorge was getting anxious about the toast he had agreed to make at his cousin's wedding. He was pleased with the content he had worked hard on. He had practiced the speech in front of his bathroom mirror. Yet he was still worried that his mind could go blank in the moment and he'd have to sit down or even leave. Recently he had bowed out of leading a meeting at the last second and asked his colleague to take over. His heart had been racing, his mouth felt as dry as a desert, and he thought he might pass out. His colleague kindly rescued him, but he was worried about what his boss might be thinking about his leadership abilities.

One night Ryan was out walking in the dark when he came across a small group of young men. They seemed interested in talking to him, but he immediately became frightened and felt panicky. He thought they looked threatening. Agitation quickly grew to a boiling point, and he suddenly found himself yelling at them. Doing an about-face to walk the other way, he pulled his hood down and tried to make himself look bigger, then turned to look back and scowled at them, waving a fist. Fearing they would follow him and he'd lose control and try to hit them, he crossed the street and took refuge in a coffee shop until they moved on.

Introducing the Stress Response

To live well with social anxiety, it is important to understand what is happening in your body. Both Jorge and Ryan had strong physical reactions to a social situation, even though Jorge perceived an interpersonal threat and Ryan a physical one. When we perceive danger, our body quickly tries its best to keep us safe. The key word here is *perceive*—we can react to situations that are not dangerous at all just as we would situations that are life-threatening. To protect us from a perceived threat, the body boosts our alertness and our ability to react quickly. We may swerve out of the way of an oncoming car or automatically duck if an object is about to fall on our head. Or we may avoid taking chances or run away from a person we think will be aggressive. Our body doesn't know the difference between real and perceived threats—it reacts exactly the same way to each. Remember that social threat can be real or perceived as well, and that our bodies react exactly the same way as when we encounter a physical danger. People who are socially anxious perceive many social interactions as potentially threatening.

Fight, Flight, or Freeze

The mechanism at work here is known as the *fight or flight* or sometimes the *freeze* response. This response to stress originates in our nervous system, which is divided into the central and autonomic nervous systems. The central nervous system includes the brain and spinal column. The autonomic nervous system is further divided into the sympathetic and parasympathetic systems. The sympathetic system prepares you to stay safe by fighting, fleeing, or freezing, depending on the situation that you are in and how you view it. You might prepare to fight an enemy or wild animal, flee an oncoming tidal wave or interpersonal conflict, or freeze so you're less visible to predators or judgmental people. These reactions are unplanned, involuntary, automatic, and often feel uncomfortable.

Your heart speeds up and sends blood to your limbs, your breathing quickens, you sweat, and your muscles tense. While it may not be obvious, your bloodstream fills with adrenaline, and your pupils dilate.

These physical changes prepare your body for immediate action. Mean-while, digestion slows down to conserve energy and glucose is released by the liver to create more energy. All human beings are equipped with this stress response.

A lesser-known and somewhat less-immediate response during a crisis is called *tend and befriend.* This response is more commonly seen among women, who may react by connecting to and trying to assist other people. It does not occur with such immediacy as the stress response but certainly can lead to healthy and helpful reactions. When I hear the term *tend and befriend,* I think of the inclination to provide food to people after a serious illness or death strikes the family.

When you perceive that you are in a threatening situation, your attention becomes hyperfocused on whatever the threat is. To under-stand how the stress response operates, think of a time when you were in danger—perhaps when your car started to slide into oncoming traf-fic while you were driving in a snowstorm. Or when you were sound asleep and the phone rang in the middle of the night. Your response would be further elevated if the phone rang while a family member was in the hospital. The startle response that is your pounding heart when the phone wakes you up is your sympathetic nervous system in action. You suddenly feel awake and in fact hyperalert.

Now think about a time when you were surprised or called on sud-denly to do something you weren't prepared for. Or picture yourself at a concert you were really looking forward to, and on which you spent a lot of money to get a front-row seat, when suddenly the lead singer asks for audience participation and singles you out to come on stage to be a backup singer (and dancer)! But you've always avoided performing in front of others because doing so makes you very anxious. It's very likely in this case that the stress response will kick in. I know that mine would! On the other hand, if the request was for the person sitting next to you, you would breathe a sigh of relief.

Emotions Involved in the Stress Response

People vary in how responsive their body is to perceived stress and how they interpret situations. You may be more reactive physiologi-cally and primed to be anxious. You may feel emotions more intensely than others—there is no way to know for sure. The emotions involved in the stress response include fear and anxiety. While these terms are often used interchangeably, they're not the same thing. Understanding the distinction can help you see how your own stress response may unfold.

FEAR VERSUS ANXIETY

Fear is your immediate physical response to perceived danger. *Anxiety* is your overall emotional state. Anxiety can arise after fear or independently of fear. It typically consists of the immediate feeling of anxiety as well as the ensuing thoughts about the feeling, the situation, and your responses. While it is usually less intense than fear, it lasts longer and includes many other feelings that can occur at the same time. It's a bit like saying "I'm nervous" rather than "I'm scared."

The physical reactions related to fear happen immediately. Anxiety arises and develops over time as thoughts and interpretations of feared situations combine with physical reactions. Long-term anxiety can also lead to the health detriments of chronic stress. Intense physical reactions, whether from fear or anxiety, may lead to panic attacks.

PANIC ATTACKS

In a scary situation, have you ever:

- ❑ Experienced an intense sudden surge of terror?
- ❑ Feared that you were going to lose control or were "going crazy"?
- ❑ Thought you were about to throw up?
- ❑ Started shaking or felt tingly?
- ❑ Felt dizzy, lightheaded, or like you might pass out?

If you have experienced these signs of a panic attack, you will know it! Panic attacks are the alert system on overdrive and are hard to miss. People with social anxiety may experience panic attacks, although panic attacks are also common in people without any mental health diagnoses and those with any number of other conditions, particularly panic disorder. Panic attacks by themselves do not indicate a diagnosable mental disorder.

A panic attack is a sudden surge of the sympathetic nervous system when you are scared. It can come on in situations in which you're suddenly frightened but that other people might consider harmless. It can happen "out of the blue" and have a very quick onset. Although panic attacks usually don't last very long, they may feel endless.

In addition to the physical signs of fear noted above (racing heart, sweating, physical tension), you may feel dizzy, lightheaded, and have a sense of impending doom as though something truly terrible is about to happen. People in a panicked state might hyperventilate or breathe very quickly. People sometimes report a sense of unreality or feeling like they are outside of their body watching themselves. Because their feelings seem inexplicable and out of the ordinary, they may think "I'm going crazy" or "I'm going to make a fool of myself" or "I'm having a heart attack." Panic attacks are a very common reason for visiting an emergency room because they feel urgent and dangerous.

If you have social anxiety, you may not experience panic attacks but you probably do experience heightened physical responses to fear. Unfortunately, there is such a thing as panic disorder, which is essentially "panic about panic." When you panic about the prospect of having a panic attack, you can start to avoid social situations in a way that is harmful to your quality of life. If you are already socially anxious, this is yet another reason to avoid!

Don't Be Tricked by Your Body

When you have social anxiety, you could have panic attacks before, during, or after social situations. Dreading these attacks can make you steer clear of situations and events you value. Imagine for a moment that you are standing at the back of a ballroom dance class. You have signed up to learn the waltz as your wedding is coming up; however, you are terrified of performing in front of others. Suddenly the instructor singles you out and takes you to the middle of the dance floor to teach you a skill to demonstrate to the class of 30 people. You are taken by surprise and have a mild panic attack. When asked to do something publicly, people with social anxiety often feel put on the spot, unprepared, and powerless to do anything about it.

Panic attacks are physically harmless, despite what your body might be telling you, but feel very distressing. You may find it hard to believe, considering the intense physical symptoms, that what is happening is "just" anxiety. Yet it's true: Panic attacks and anxiety attacks are one and the same. Like Jorge when he skipped out on leading a meeting, you may find yourself escaping from situations in which you feel anxiety building, for fear that you'll have a full-blown panic attack. Panic attacks can certainly have negative consequences that you'd prefer to elude.

Sometimes people fear losing control of their bodily functions during a panic attack—trembling or visibly shaking, blushing, vomiting, or even losing bladder or bowel control. These thoughts are related to the fear of being embarrassed and becoming the center of attention. While it's very rare to lose control of these bodily functions, the fear of embarrassment if it did occur can be powerful. Some people are less anxious about these fears when they know that a bathroom is readily available and may use a toilet finder app (like Gottago). Heightened muscle tension can lead to trembling, just as increased blood flow can lead to blushing and gastrointestinal changes can lead to nausea. All of the potential changes are related to the physiological response to fear in your body and are temporary and harmless.

> Panic attacks will not hurt you. Changing your behavior out of fear of panic attacks can have negative consequences.

Pulling Apart the Fear Response to Take Control

In general, the more intense your response is to a perceived threat, the more difficult it is to figure out what to do other than fight, flee, or freeze. Think of anger and how quickly situations can get out of control and lead to fighting and aggression. People can also respond intensely when exciting and positive things happen as well. Anger may lead to an urge to attack, sadness may lead to an urge to withdraw, and anxiety may lead to an urge to avoid. During all these situations, your mind will be keenly focused on the immediate situation and on reducing the uncomfortable emotion. Your primary urge will be to reduce the emotion rather than solve the problem that raised it—even though the latter is the better solution. Intense emotion interferes with your ability to think clearly. Just as it's not a good idea to make big decisions in the midst of a crisis, the middle of a panic attack is not a good time to solve a problem. *Figure out how to feel better before trying to solve any problems.*

Figuring out how to feel better starts with understanding where you can interrupt the fear response. Think of your own fear response:

- What physical signs do you usually notice? What happens first?
- Do you have one particularly sensitive bodily reaction? Some people tend to notice a racing heart, whereas others may become hot and sweaty.
- In what situations have you noticed these signs?
- Do you see any pattern to these situations?
- Have you paid attention to how long these physical signs lasted?
- Are you able to identify the emotion that you are experiencing when your body is reacting?
- Have you tried to do anything to reduce or change your response?
- Have you been distressed by your response and tried to hide it?
- What thoughts or ideas do you have about not being able to control your initial fear?

Numerous steps can be taken to help manage these reactions when they occur and are distressing. In many situations, you can quickly deescalate these responses, which then leads to more planful thinking and problem solving.

Strategies to Manage Intense Reactions

Most people who have experienced high levels of anxiety are told to "relax" or take up mindfulness meditation. Relaxation is intended to help reduce the reactivity of your mind and body and produce a calm state of being, whereas mindfulness is intended to help with acceptance and tolerance of whatever you are experiencing. Overall, I certainly recommend these types of coping skills as they may reduce your overall stress level, but they can be difficult to engage in the middle of a difficult situation when you need them the most. If you are at a podium, you might be able to pause and take a deep breath, but you are not going to lie down for a 20-minute relaxation session!

A better first step is to do something to notice when your reactions are occurring. Try **STOP:**

- **S**top
- **T**ake a breath
- **O**bserve carefully
- **P**roceed with awareness

This easy-to-remember process reminds us to slow down and consider what to do next.

The following strategies are intended to be used for strong physical responses—panic as well as other intense reactions related to fight, flight, or freeze—in the moment.

Strategies to Counteract the Physical Response

Any of the following will change your response and ground your body in the present moment. Essentially, you are countering a strong response with another strong but different response. Try any of the following right now:

- Stamp your feet firmly on the floor, one at a time. Repeat five times.

- Clench your fists and hold the tightness for 5 seconds. Now release and notice the difference. Repeat five times.
- Do five jumping jacks or, if you practice yoga and can, get on the floor and do a plank and hold it for 30 seconds.

Stamping your feet is an immediate reminder of the ground or floor under your feet. An activity requiring focus and muscle control counteracts the adrenaline in your body and will usually help you pay attention to something else. It provides an alternative explanation to how you feel, as you will attribute your racing heart to jumping up and down rather than anxiety. Obviously, you will not be able to use most of these in a social situation unless you are in a gym or go into another physical space.

Strategies to Shift to a Different Physical Sensation

- **Use cold.** Go into a bathroom and splash cold water on your face—it will be bracing and give you an immediate jolt. If you have a glass of water with ice cubes in it, take out an ice cube and put it on your wrist for a minute. This strategy can be used in many social situations if you put your wrists under the table.

- **Use taste.** Carry some very sour candies in your bag and put one in your mouth or eat some spicy food if you are out for a meal. Your attention will immediately focus on the temperature or taste and will shift. The jolt to your taste buds also wakes you up! I have a client who keeps very sour candies in her car for instances of road rage. Some of these candies are not for the faint of heart (ratings of the extreme sourness are available online). Both ice cubes and small candies are reasonably convenient to try in many situations.

- **While standing, shake both of your hands vigorously a few times.** Similarly to the physical intensity exercises above, you will focus on the blood flow into your hands and experience a different sensation.

Change Your Environment

In many instances, it's appropriate to change locations. Go into a hallway or a different room to catch your breath. It's always okay to use the washroom and try some of the preceding strategies there. If you're indoors, go outdoors. The simple act of moving and changing spaces can help reduce or change your reactions.

Strategies to Use When You Can't Move Around

It may be difficult or even impossible to get up and move in certain situations, and you may not have access to food or candy. For example, if you are in a job interview, out for dinner, or talking to another passenger on an airplane, it would be awkward or impossible to start doing jumping jacks! Here are some other options:

• **Pause.** Remember that if you are asked a question, an immediate response is not necessarily required. Try pausing, taking a breath, and saying something like "Can you give me a moment?" or "Can you repeat the question?" or "Can you elaborate on the question?"

• **Answer the question for which you have an answer ready.** This response shows you know something, buys you some time, and forces the other person to clarify what they really want you to talk about! These latter ideas are favorites for students in oral examinations. Notice how politicians often repeat questions or duck them completely!

• **Refuse the person's request.** If you are suddenly asked to do something in public that you didn't expect, say "No, thanks" firmly and politely. Those with social anxiety are often eager to please others and do things that they didn't want or intend to say yes to. If it's difficult to say no, it might be easier to say "I'll think about it and get back to you later." If you're asked to go onstage and you have performance anxiety, say no!

• **Change your focus from inside yourself to outside yourself.** Really look around and notice your environment. Mindfulness meditation has many different exercises that can be helpful for shifting focus. A mindfulness exercise such as 5-4-3-2-1 can help. Focus upon five things you see, four things you hear, three things you can touch, two things you can smell, and one you can taste. Note that all five senses are used in this exercise and that the task requires close attention to what is going on, which distracts you from your thoughts by increasing your focus on sensations. If you happen to be in a place with low light and lots of sounds or smells, change the order. It can even be done with eyes closed; just put the vision part lower down the list (for example, focus on two things rather than five things that you can see, which includes any light, which usually can be experienced with eyes closed). To become adept at using 5-4-3-2-1, consider practicing the sequence when you have a little free time and are not feeling anxious.

• **Breathe slowly and deeply.** We're often told to try deep breathing when anxious. The problem is that often we end up breathing both more deeply and too quickly. It's easy to breathe quickly when anxious. People experiencing panic attacks sometimes hyperventilate, leading them to feel dizzy and lightheaded. So, if appropriate and if you are not expected to talk, try counting to help you breathe both deeply and slowly. Breathe in to a slow count of four and then out to a slow count of four; then use six and even eight counts. It may help to try what is called *box breathing.* Picture a square or box and breathe in to a count of four (side 1), hold for a count of four (side 2), breathe out for a count of four (side 3), and then hold for a final count of four (side 4). The four steps remind you to hold and not breathe quickly. Usually, it will clear your mind and help increase a sense of calmness and relaxation in your body. Sometimes it's helpful to repeat once every hour or so during a stressful day.

• **Label your physiological response *body noise.*** Some bodies are more responsive to threat than others. One of my colleagues uses the phrase *body noise* to describe this phenomenon—the "noise" being the physiological response your body generates to get your attention. The phrase is neutral, in contrast with words like *fear, panic, anger,* and *stress,* which have negative connotations. Relabeling the responses as body noise can help create some distance and an attitude of observation. My colleague even went on to foster an attitude of interest in the sensations rather than anxiety about them. "My body is noisy right now. I notice that my heart is beating rapidly. I wonder what will happen next and why this is happening right now." If we notice our body's response and pay attention in a neutral and curious way, we are less likely to be frightened or reactive and have negative thoughts about it.

• **Learn to ride the wave of sensations.** It's important to remember that the physical signs of a panic attack typically begin suddenly, rise to a crest, and then gradually dissipate. They always reduce in intensity, usually quite quickly. This reduction happens because it is not possible for your body to remain in such a heightened state indefinitely—it will wear itself out, and it's exhausting. I recently heard someone describe this strategy as letting your reactions in the front door and letting them go through the house and out the back door but not stopping and inviting them to stay for tea.

• **Try timing the panic as well as rating it on a scale from 1 to 100.** Most people believe that the panic sensations last longer than they actually do. Rating the intensity of sensations demonstrates that there is a range, rather than assuming it's always 100/100. Learning the variability and timing of the sensations helps create distance and a sense of control.

Beware of Negative Strategies That Could Be Harmful Rather Than Helpful

It's common for people with intense reactions to look for substances like drugs or alcohol that might help them feel better. Not only can these be harmful over the long term, but they are usually not effective in the short term as they inhibit other coping strategies. Prescription drugs such as those that reduce anxiety (such as Ativan) may help reduce physiological sensations but can be habit forming and also harmful in the long term. They can often become a kind of avoidance strategy, which can maintain your fear and keep you anxious. People who use substances to manage their anxiety may be able to go ahead and do what they are frightened of, but they've given away the credit for managing their anxiety to the drug. They may say things like "I couldn't have done it without having that drink," which leaves their coping skills unimproved. It's easy to depend on something or someone else to cope rather than learning skills that increase confidence and a sense of self-efficacy.

Claire was very shy and reluctant to try new activities. She had a few friends who goaded her when she went out with them after her university classes. One time, they met up before going to a party and "pre-drinking" was suggested. After several quick rounds of rowdy shots, Claire started to feel lightheaded but braver. They all went to the party and she had a good time. The next time shots were suggested she was up for it, and pre-drinking started to become a regular occurrence. She developed a belief that she couldn't manage without the alcohol.

Other strategies besides drugs or alcohol may also be harmful. I have had clients who fear certain body reactions (such as sudden urges to use the washroom) limit their fluid or food intake. While these strategies are not likely to be harmful if used occasionally, they could be dangerous if you were in a sporting event such as marathon or on a lengthy plane trip. People who worry a lot about sweating or trembling may try to mask these signs, inadvertently worsening the problem. For example, wearing extra clothing to hide sweat stains will certainly make a person sweat more and look a bit unusual.

Jorge decided that he would go ahead and agree to give the toast to the groom at the wedding. He really wanted to honor his cousin and thought that his speech was funny and clever. He practiced giving it several times to his family, while sitting down and then standing up. He tried it with a makeshift podium, which helped give him a place to put his notes. He had thoughts such as "the podium will hide my shaking knees and part of my body." It helped that he practiced in a similar situation.

The morning of the wedding day, he checked out the actual setting. He stood at the front of the room and visualized the audience. These steps were helpful, although he remained anxious for most of the day. When the time came and he was introduced, he stood up and walked slowly to the podium. He paused, took out his notes, and took several slow breaths to calm his body. He told himself that it was okay not to be perfect—no one is, and it's important to make the effort. He had a glass of water at the ready in case his mouth became dry. He started the talk and made a few early small mistakes (in his mind anyway; no one else seemed to notice). He spoke a bit quickly, but a few moments in, his anxiety started to reduce and he was able to slow down, take some pauses, and scan the room. It was helpful to look around and not focus on any one person. Once he was done and raised his wine glass to give the toast, he noticed that his hand was trembling somewhat, but he did not spill anything, so it wasn't a big deal. People laughed at his jokes and clapped when he was done!

Strategies to Manage Your Emotional Reactions

Lisa was out riding her bike one evening after dinner. She was an experienced cyclist and always wore a helmet. She had a repair kit on her bike as well as her cell phone in her pocket in case she needed to contact someone. That evening it began raining heavily. Lisa skidded while going around a corner and hit a bump, which sent her flying over the handlebars. She landed quite hard and took a few minutes to sort herself out but did not feel scared. She did not hit her head or do any significant damage. She was prepared to look after herself. Another cyclist stopped to help. At that point Lisa became uncomfortable and self-conscious. She hated asking for help and feeling vulnerable in front of others. She jumped up, got on her bike, and quickly rode away without saying a word. She waved her hand at the other person, who was a bit confused about what had just happened.

In this situation the person stopping to help Lisa led her to feel more anxiety than the fall itself. Her thoughts had a chance to kick in, and she felt weak and embarrassed. She began to have thoughts that he would think she was stupid, irresponsible, or even worse, helpless. Those thoughts led to her leaving quickly and not saying thank you. Many people with social anxiety prefer to be left alone rather than being viewed as needing help. How would you react in this situation? Would you be likely to ask for help?

• **Remember that emotions are related to how you view the situation rather than the situation itself.** They occur in conjunction with an interpretation of an event. They are complicated by lots of different factors, including the meaning of the event. For Lisa, falling could mean that she wasn't a good cyclist, that she wasn't taking appropriate precautions, and that she couldn't take care of herself.

Those thoughts led to feelings of embarrassment and could also have led to guilt, shame, or other complicated emotions.

• **Keep in mind that anxiety is a consequence of overestimating the risk involved in a situation and underestimating one's coping abilities.** For people with social anxiety, the risk is usually interpersonal. Lisa had a good sense of her cycling skills and preparation and was able to assess the physical risks as low as she did not seem hurt. Consequently, her anxiety was low after her fall. When the other cyclist stopped, this immediately changed as she overestimated the risks (being judged) and underestimated her coping skills (being able to talk to the other person, to accept or decline an offer of help). Her anxiety rose, and she rode away. Then she felt additional anxiety over the circumstances of her "escape" from the social consequences of the fall.

• **Know that shame is deeper and more complicated than embarrassment.** The emotional response of shame is complex. You don't just feel embarrassed about something you've done, but about who you are at your core and your being unworthy of love or attention. It's the perception of having done something deeply inappropriate, immoral, or wrong. It may lead to a response where you just want to disappear and hide what you've done. Lisa may place moral value on independence, being in control and always able to help herself. People who struggle with accepting help often place more value on independence than the average person, and dislike appearing needy. Some people have had deeply shaming experiences during childhood or adolescence where they were humiliated for some central aspect of their sense of self (such as weight, appearance, gender, intellect). Lisa may have a history of being shamed as a child for not being able to do everything for herself.

• **Remember that most people experience numerous emotions at the same time.** People experience many emotions—they can happen very quickly and change quickly as well, depending on the evolving situation. They can be intense or mild.

• **Practice awareness of your emotions.** *Say the words out loud.* Many people struggle with knowing how they feel. The easy ones are *mad, sad,* and *glad.* Remember that *okay, good, bad,* and *busy* are not emotions. If you generally respond with one of those four words when asked how you are feeling, try an experiment for a few days where you substitute different words. These could be *tired* or *hungry,* as it is easier to be aware of the state of your body than your emotions. Have you ever used the word *hangry*? People who are hungry often get a bit irritated and impatient by the feeling, as many parents know. It may be a surprise when a snack is seen as a cure for anger! Once you have done the experiment, try including some emotion-related words, such as *cheerful, happy, overwhelmed,* or *confused.* With practice, you will gradually increase both your emotional vocabulary and your awareness. It helps to say the words out loud.

• **Recognize that it's okay to be okay!** People also don't go through their lives experiencing intense emotions all the time—that would be exhausting! I suspect that someone has asked you how you feel and you have said "okay." While "okay" is not a feeling, you probably weren't hiding anything; you were just feeling relatively neutral. It can be difficult if you're put on the spot and asked to describe your feelings and not much comes to mind! Very quickly, you could begin to feel a bit irritated with the question.

Moving Forward

This chapter has discussed what happens in our bodies when fear is activated by some type of trigger. Fear is not the same as anxiety. Its function is protective, and our bodies react with the fight, flight, or freeze response that happens almost instantaneously. It can take us by surprise and feel overwhelming, leading us to be unable to think clearly. Some people experience panic attacks or other very intense reactions, which is our body in a kind of overdrive. It is important to see these reactions as uncomfortable and distressing but not dangerous. To live your best life alongside social anxiety, it's important to understand that these reactions can be informative rather than scary.

There are many different ways in which to manage our body's reactions to perceived threats—first remember the **STOP** acronym.

Slow down and respond rather than react. There are many helpful strategies to learn and practice. It's important to be aware that some strategies to reduce fear can be unhealthy, such as substance abuse, avoidance, or making sudden big decisions, like leaving a job or relationship. The first step is to manage your reactions and reduce their intensity before doing anything else. Our feelings are very much mediated by how we think about the situation, and in the next chapter you'll gain understanding and strategies for managing the thoughts that hurt you or get in the way.

5

how to get to the root of it all— your thoughts

Your mind plays a vital role in social anxiety: It can keep you anxious or depressed, or it can help you feel better and move on with your life. The core symptoms of social anxiety are thoughts—the fear of negative evaluation or being judged harshly by other people. Negative thoughts are sometimes called *maladaptive, distorted,* or *dysfunctional,* but these terms sound disparaging. So I sometimes just use the terms *unhelpful, hurtful,* or simply *thoughts that get in the way.* A client once said "Not only do I feel terrible, but you're telling me that my thoughts are all wrong?" At that point, we came up with some other words to describe her thoughts.

The root of social anxiety is worry about what other people think of you. While almost all of us want to be liked and thought well of by others, if you have social anxiety these thoughts tend to dominate your life and create distractions and obstacles to living well. The way in which we think affects how we feel and what we do. We can convince ourselves to do things or not to do things, that people like us or hate us, that our social skills are perfectly fine, adequate, or absolutely dreadful. These thoughts may be accurate at times, but for socially anxious people they are often distorted and hurtful. Most people with social anxiety disorder view themselves in unfavorable ways and make negative predictions about how they will act, what they may say, and what will occur in upcoming situations. These thoughts tend to happen quickly and automatically and are heightened when you're anxious.

What Are Thoughts Made Up Of?

Amira was trying unsuccessfully to get to sleep. She had to get up early to drive her mother to a doctor's appointment. She was upset with herself because once again she had agreed to take her, as her brother claimed that he had an important work meeting. Amira did not stand up for herself and say no since she was currently out of work and did not think she had anything important to do. Her thoughts were "I'm being taken advantage of," "I'm a doormat," "I'll never amount to anything," and "My mother idolizes my brother and takes me for granted." Her feelings were frustration, anger, and anxiety that she would not be able to get to sleep. She was very tired, and her thoughts kept coming and coming like a tornado. She started having memories of times when her brother won sports competitions in school while she sat on the sidelines or when her mother told her about something he had said as if it was a fact and Amira's opinions didn't count. She began feeling agitated and was tossing and turning until she reached for her phone and started scrolling through her social media feeds. She finally fell asleep at 2:30 and woke up groggy and cranky the next day.

Both how Amira was thinking and what she was thinking interfered with her ability to fall asleep. Her thoughts came rapidly, with one thought leading to another. She was unable to shift this process. This is the *how,* or the process of thinking. Her negative thoughts ("I'm a doormat") are the *what,* or the content of negative thoughts resulting in frustration and agitation.

Essentially, taking charge of how you think and what you think is important for living well with social anxiety. Let's start with the how.

How We Think: The Process

Many of us have lain awake at night with our mind in a whirlwind, running over and over something we did or didn't say. These types of worries, whether accurate or inaccurate, can be a big concern for anyone who is anxious. People with anxiety sometimes describe these types of thoughts as similar to being on a treadmill with no way to get off or a hamster wheel of the mind. They can seem like an endless loop that is difficult to interrupt.

Our minds tend to be busy places. According to research, the average person has about 60,000 thoughts each and every day! Thoughts both describe what is going on around us and provide a running dialogue and commentary. It is not natural to step back and really listen to them. One thought typically leads to another to another and another, and each may be only remotely related to the original thought, much like the telephone game you may have played as a child, where a whispered sentence passed around a circle is wildly distorted by the time the last player has heard it.

Our internal dialogue can feel cluttered and anxiety provoking or sometimes just distracting. Much of the time, we don't notice it at all. But have you ever been kept awake at night because you suddenly thought of something that you had to do the next day? Or been distracted while driving because of something you forgot to say to someone? Our thoughts can be quite intrusive, particularly when we're anxious. And for people who are socially anxious, many of these thoughts focus on negative judgment and are difficult to counterbalance.

Trying to stop intrusive thoughts tends to be an ineffective and counterproductive strategy because the mind abhors a vacuum and works hard to find something to think about. Practitioners of some forms of meditation are able to keep their thoughts from hijacking their mind, but not by trying to push them out and leaving a void. *Your mind cannot be a blank space.*

Strategies to Calm Your Intrusive Thoughts

To calm your mind you need to shift the content of your thoughts. But that means slowing down the process first. You can't create a blank mind, but there are some strategies that can change the process of thinking:

- **Write it down.** In Chapter 2 you learned how to monitor your thoughts and probably found that getting them out of your head and onto paper was helpful. While whirling busy thoughts may be difficult to catch, writing them down on a self-monitoring form on paper or a digital device will lead to more awareness and slow them down.

- **Get out of your head.** Deliberately focus your attention on something different, like an everyday task that requires some but not too much attention—think folding laundry, cleaning up your email inbox, or weeding your garden. Many people suggest going for a walk or listening to music as diversions. But unless you're doing a challenging hike or attending to the details of the music, these strategies often don't take up enough of your attention to stop you from worrying. So choose a task that requires some focus.

- **Try mental puttering #1: Visualize a space you know well.** For example, visualize in great detail the home you grew up in or any other space that isn't stressful or emotionally charged for you— your local supermarket (ensure that you mentally pick up the produce to check for ripeness!), a family cottage, or a favorite campsite. If it's a former home, enter the front door and look at each detail in turn, such as what is on the floor and the pictures on the walls. Open the front closet, look at the light fixture and the ceiling, and then go from room to room in a slow, methodical fashion. In your mind, open the kitchen cupboard doors to see what is inside. This task can be surprisingly difficult to do.

- **Try mental puttering #2: Picture yourself doing a physical task in detail.** Visualize yourself skiing, hiking, or doing a dance routine. Feel all of the steps and shifts in your body, including the flexing of your muscles and changes in position, as well as the temperature, the feel of the snow, a glint of sunlight or the sound of music. If your worries return, gently push them aside and tell yourself that you'll deal with them later. Return to your image and remind yourself that it is natural for minds to wander from one thing to another.

- **Do something different that will shift your emotional state.** Watch a funny episode of a sitcom that you enjoy or play a video game that you like. Listen to a funny podcast. Once your emotional state changes even a bit, the thoughts will seem less important and are likely to dissipate. Thoughts and feelings are closely connected, and when one changes, usually the other will as well.

• **Distance your thoughts.** View them from afar, reminding yourself that they are "mental events" and will diminish and change with time. See your thoughts written on a screen or hear them spoken by a famous person. Say them in a funny voice or very, very slowly. The tone will shift, and your perspective will likely be changed as well.

• **Shift the environment or change the scene.** If you are in bed and your thoughts are buzzing and you cannot fall asleep, get out of bed and go into another room even if it's just for 10 minutes. If you're sitting at your desk and having looping thoughts about an upcoming difficult task, get up and do some stretches. A change of scene sometimes will help shift your thoughts. Even standing up and moving around can be helpful. Any change can help. You may notice that this strategy was suggested in Chapter 4 for helping reduce the intensity of emotions. While thoughts are whirling, emotions tend to be strong as well.

• **Thought stopping does not work.** Deliberate efforts to stop your thoughts are likely to backfire. Years ago, psychologists used to recommend what was called *thought stopping*, which involved simply telling yourself to "Stop it" and snapping an elastic band on your wrist. Not only is this strategy ineffective, but it can backfire and actually increase the negative thoughts. Trying really hard not to think of something often makes it difficult to think of anything else! It is far more effective to gently shift your thoughts to something else.

PRACTICE EXERCISE 1: Thoughts can't be banished

Close your eyes and try to relax. You have been feeling stressed and want to shift your thoughts. Try to create a blank space in your mind. Instead of a void opening up, imagine that suddenly a pink elephant bounces into view. Then you see groups of them happily bouncing around. They keep popping unbidden into your mind. For the next 60 seconds (set a timer on your phone or watch), do not think of pink elephants. Work really, really hard not to have these images in your mind. No matter what you do, stop these images from coming. Take the images away and replace them with nothing—just a blank mind.

What happened? In most cases the harder you try to banish a thought, the more it persists.

The preceding strategies and practice exercise illustrate that when you want to slow down intrusive, bothersome thoughts, you're better off replacing them with something else. But learning to do this focuses only on the how of thoughts, not the what.

What We Think About: The Content

There is a great deal of content in our busy minds, and much of it arises automatically—quickly and without intention. *Automatic thoughts* are about various topics: what we've done, are doing, and have to do; ourselves, others, the situation we're in, the world around us; how we feel, physically, mentally, and emotionally.

Where do these automatic thoughts come from? They are the product of your underlying beliefs, your values, your history, the situation you're in, and your interpretation of all of these factors. You may or may not be aware of them, but some automatic thoughts are common among socially anxious people. Here are examples:

- I won't be able to think of anything to say and will look stupid.
- Everyone is looking at me and knows that I'm terribly anxious as I'm blushing.
- I will look awkward, and my voice will crack if I talk.
- I'm boring, dull, and unlikable.
- I'm not worth talking to; others might as well ignore me.
- Other people are not trustworthy and are quick to judge.
- Anxiety is a sign of weakness, and it's awful to be full of fear.

- Others are successful, skilled, funny, and friendly.
- I made a fool of myself the other day. I'm terrified to go back there again.
- I might as well stay home and give up. I'm such a loser.
- I am defective at the core.

Recognizing such patterns can help you shift away from them and improve the quality of your life. *The essential symptom of social anxiety is thoughts about negative social judgment, and other symptoms grow from that root.* Fears about offending others, being embarrassed and humiliated, or showing emotional vulnerability in front of others and being judged can all lead to great discomfort and attempts to avoid this discomfort. It's perfectly normal to try to avoid this discomfort. It's the anxiety that leads to lots of other emotions such as guilt, irritability, sadness, embarrassment, and shame. The discomfort also leads to being quiet, attempting to fade into the background, or leaving and becoming socially isolated. Some people who are socially anxious appear irritable without necessarily intending to. Others with social anxiety appear disinterested or snobbish. Any of these patterns of negative thoughts are followed by anxious feelings and behaviors and have negative consequences for life. So it's important to examine your thought patterns for accuracy and also determine where they come from if you want to make a change in your social anxiety.

Could What You Think Come from Your Biases?

You may be aware of your negative thoughts but believe they are true. All human beings, however, are biased in their thinking patterns. Computer systems are much more logical and predictable than people (but less creative and interesting!). If the same data goes into a computer program 10 times, the program will always come up with the same "correct" answer. In contrast, if 10 people witness the same motor vehicle accident, they will recall 10 slightly different versions of the same event. If 10 people are at the same social event, all their experiences will be quite different from each other. A very important point is that your thoughts are not facts. They are your interpretation of what you see and think about. People don't have thoughts that they believe to be wrong or biased—that wouldn't make sense.

> Don't believe everything you think!
> It's just your opinion!

We All Wear Different Glasses: Our Mental Filters

We all tend to think we're right most of the time, although people who are socially anxious are likely to put more value in others' opinions than their own. Even though everyone has their own point of view and sees the world "through their own glasses," it's easy to assume that others see things the same way we do. People who view themselves negatively will conclude that others view them negatively as well. If you think others are looking at you and drawing negative conclusions, you might not check it out but just assume it is true.

Sometimes we call these metaphorical glasses *mental filters*. Some people wear rose-colored glasses and see the world in a positive light. Others have glasses that create a negative light (perhaps blue). Still others may see the world in a distorted or skewed way. Another metaphor that is sometimes used is that our mental filters are just like light filters; they allow certain experiences and events into our awareness but block out or filter others. We see only what we permit ourselves to see but usually don't realize that the filters are even present. This tendency is sometimes called *confirmation bias*—we will see what confirms the biases we already have.

Are Your Thoughts Driven by Superstitions?

Have you ever bought a lottery ticket? Millions of people do every day, hoping to be the one who wins a million dollars. To buy such a ticket is a sign of unrealistic hope, as the chances of winning are very poor. People do lots of things to increase their luck in different circumstances, such as choose a lucky number or carry a rabbit's foot. Cultures around the world have certain customs to increase good luck or decrease bad. Many of these customs go back centuries, such as throwing salt over one's left shoulder or having protection against the evil eye. Do you use any of these tricks? While harmless, they are signs of superstitious thinking. On the plus side, you might feel more confident and less anxious if you have a certain piece of "lucky" jewelry or clothing on. If it makes you feel better, you are more likely to try new things.

Harmful Thoughts Involving Biases

Our thoughts can be accurate or inaccurate, in negative or positive ways. How do we figure out which we're experiencing and how it's contributing to social anxiety? One way is to examine our thoughts for "cognitive distortions." Many books written about cognitive-behavioral therapy include lists of different ways our thoughts are distorted, and you may have encountered some of them. But the terms used can be confusing, even for me although I have worked in the field for many years. So here you'll read instead about the main types of harmful thinking. All of them involve biases that lead to feeling bad about yourself.

FUTURE-ORIENTED THOUGHTS

Often harmful thoughts are all about the future. Negative predictions about the future or what will happen when others think a certain way occur in all anxious people. These predictions can be called *catastrophic thinking, fortune telling,* or *jumping to conclusions.* We like to think that we are accurate, but we often are incorrect. Remember that if something hasn't happened, it's impossible to know if our predictions will come true. Everything regarding the future is unknown, even the immediate future! Do you remember (if you're old enough) the "Y2K" fears of 1999, and the panic in some quarters about the beginning of the new millennium? People prepared for the worst. In early 2020, we may have worried about many potential catastrophic events, such as global warming, wars, or the state of the economy, but few people were concerned about an impending pandemic. Often what we worry about does not happen and what we didn't think to worry about does!

It's easy to jump to conclusions without getting the facts straight. It's only human to work hard to understand the world around us and the people in it. Making predictions about the future helps us feel more in control but can also lead to intense fear ("I shouldn't go on that trip as the airplane will crash"). Positive predictions can also lead to unwarranted excitement ("I am certain to win the lottery"). When I was a young student, I had a boss who bought lottery tickets and spent much of his day planning where he would go on vacation with his winnings. Maps of the world were strewn on his desk. He not only didn't win but was let go from the job.

PAST-ORIENTED THOUGHTS

Thoughts about the past may involve regrets or self-blame. Have you ever been unable to think of what to say at a particular moment and then had thoughts afterward about what you could have said? People who are socially anxious are prone to have both negative thoughts about the future and concerns about the past. It bears repeating that "thoughts are just thoughts" and not facts.

WHY DID SOMETHING HAPPEN?

Another broad category of harmful thinking involves trying to figure out the cause of what's happening or has happened. Trying to attribute certain outcomes or events to someone (including yourself) or something can involve labeling ("I'm such a loser—it's all my fault"; "I'm stupid and will never amount to anything"; "If it weren't for my parents, I'd be fine") or blaming your own actions ("It's because of my poor planning that this trip did not work out"). It can also involve *emotional reasoning*—trying to reason from your feelings, not the other way around ("I'm scared, so this situation must be scary" rather than "This is a very scary place, so I'm frightened").

Thoughts about others may involve mind reading ("I'm sure that that person doesn't want to see me; they looked the other way when I passed them on the street") or blame ("They are so snobbish"). Mind reading is very common. We often react on the basis of what we think the other person is thinking or feeling without checking it out.

The mind can be quite creative in how it interprets what is going on and, in this way, maintain socially anxious beliefs. Once we think we have figured out what is going on, we stop looking for information that might contradict or challenge our first interpretation. When Lisa saw Jon scowling while looking in her direction, she assumed he was angry at her. Based on that interpretation, she looked down at the floor and did not see him smile when he saw her a few seconds later. He had been distracted by his own thoughts.

It is important to remember that most situations have multiple causes. Imagine that you've just been involved in a car accident. When the police arrive, you may be tempted to say "It was my fault" even though the weather, road conditions, the vehicle or tires, the other driver, distractions, as well as the driving skills of both drivers may have been involved. The reality is that almost nothing is likely to be *all* your fault. (If you had that much power, you could change the world!)

WHAT GLASSES ARE YOU WEARING?

Another category of harmful thoughts has to do with our mental filters. As noted above, we all see the world using different "filters," which means that our attention is focused on certain information while other information is neglected or missed entirely. Think of a time when you've been in a room full of people and suddenly heard your name spoken from the other side of the room. Your ears perked up, whereas you weren't paying attention to that conversation before. If you have a broken leg and are trying to navigate the world wearing a cast and using crutches, you will be alert to curbs, stairs, and physical barriers in your environment. Or if you have ever been pregnant, it suddenly seems as though the rates of pregnancy have increased as you notice pregnant people and hear pregnancy-related stories that you may not have listened to before. People who are socially anxious are particularly likely to pay attention to some types of information and neglect others.

Our minds are very different than computers, and we can draw conclusions with no evidence, minimal evidence, or inaccurate information. Because of our mental filters we may see what we expect to see and miss seeing certain things entirely as we focus on one aspect of the picture. If you believe you're uninteresting and boring, you are likely going to be hypervigilant to others looking away, yawning, and taking out their phones even if these things have nothing to do with you—and this "evidence" will reinforce your preexisting assumptions.

EXTREME THOUGHTS

You may have noticed that most of these types of thinking tend to be extreme rather than nuanced. This is sometimes referred to as *overgeneralization, black-and-white thinking,* and *all-or-none thinking.* For example, socially anxious people may use harsh labels or words that they wouldn't say out loud to anyone else ("I'm so stupid and useless"). When you are socially anxious, you may blame yourself for something that was not your fault ("That person is glaring at me because I said the wrong thing"). You may discount positive comments or interpret them in negative ways ("Joe complimented me on my new haircut because he thought I really needed one and looked terrible before").

Strategies for Feeling Better by Changing What You Think

With practice, most people can identify biases in their thinking. It can, however, be tricky to shift or change those thoughts. It's easy to be distracted by our internal dialogue, especially when the dialogue is negative or when we're feeling uncomfortable. People who make negative predictions about not being able to think of what to say next in a conversation, for example, may be mentally rehearsing a comment and then totally miss what is being said. Ironically, thinking of the next comment makes it much less likely for you to hear the conversation and respond naturally.

Fortunately, there are many ways in which to shift and reduce negative thinking patterns. The first and most important requirement is an awareness that can be obtained by slowing down and getting some distance from your thoughts. Remember that thoughts are just that: thoughts. You can evaluate your own thinking, just as you can evaluate the thoughts or ideas of others.

One effective beginning point is to write down your distressing automatic thoughts. Looking at them in black and white, either on paper or on a screen, can help you figure out their accuracy as well as your patterns. It can help you see whether these thoughts are closely linked to an emotional response. Over time, you can start to examine whether certain thoughts occur in predictable types of situations, and you can look for patterns in both the process and content of what you are saying to yourself.

> Remember that thoughts are just mental events.

LEARN TO THINK LIKE A SCIENTIST

Remember that our thoughts are mental events and may or may not be accurate. Once you are able to step back and be more aware of them, it's very helpful to question them. Here are some helpful questions to ask yourself about your thoughts:

- What is the automatic thought? The first step is to pay attention and "catch" the thought.
- Is the thought accurate? How do you know? What type of information are you paying attention to?
- What is the evidence that the thought is accurate?
- What is the evidence that the thought might not be accurate?
- What would someone else say about this thought?

It's difficult to know how accurate thoughts are without looking at the evidence, kind of like a scientist might. A scientist considers different predictions (sometimes called *hypotheses*) and then might test them out by collecting evidence or data. So, instead of assuming that your negative thought is true, you can examine the evidence for and against it.

Amira managed to wake up on time and picked her mother up to take her to her physician appointment. She was feeling irritable as she had slept poorly. When she was helping her mother up the stairs at the front of the building, her mother complained that she was holding her arm too tightly and might even leave a bruise. Amira's first thought was "I can never do anything right," and she loosened her grip on her mother's arm. When they got to the receptionist, Amira gave her mother's name without thinking, and her mother commented that she could have done it herself and didn't want to be treated like an invalid. Amira felt very upset after these comments and vowed she would insist that her brother take time off work next time to take their mother to her appointment.

Then, Amira decided to complete a chart to assess her thinking patterns:

> *Negative thought: "I never do anything right."*
>
> *Evidence to support this thought: Mother complained twice about how I was treating her this morning. I don't have a job or anything important to do.*
>
> *Evidence that does not support this thought: I was able to get up on time after a poor night's sleep, we arrived at the appointment on time, and I am generally very helpful to my mother even though she may not appreciate it.*

By doing this exercise and thinking like a scientist, Amira realized that her initial automatic thought was quite extreme, using the words "never" and "anything." She knew that in reality she generally does some things right but also makes some mistakes.

FIGURE OUT THE FACTS

It's surprisingly difficult to know exactly what is true and accurate. If Amira were having difficulty figuring out the "facts" or evidence, she could ask someone whose opinion she trusts, "Can you think of anything that I've done that is right or not wrong?" Or she might work with her initial thought "I never do anything right" to make it more specific, such as "I sometimes make mistakes in my work" or "I may be somewhat insensitive to my mother, as I'm angry that she takes me for granted." These comments are not as extreme (for example, *never* is changed to *sometimes*), and it will be easier to look at evidence for and against them. Amira could then make a list of mistakes that she had made as well as a list of times when her work had been accurate.

The chart that Amira used is shown in the exercise on page 107. It is straightforward and can be used to look at evidence for and against your thoughts.

PRACTICE EXERCISE 2: Looking at the evidence

Consider a frequent thought that you have and analyze it using the form on page 107 (also available to download and print at *www.guilford.com/dobson3-forms*).

USE LESS COLORFUL OR EVEN BORING LANGUAGE

Many negative thoughts are extreme, pejorative, and emotionally loaded, such as "I'm a bad person" or "They hate me." With intense emotions come intense thoughts and vice versa. Some of these thoughts are bossy and judgmental. For example, any thought that starts out as "I should" or "I never" or "I always" is very likely inaccurate as people are seldom one way 100% of the time. Shift some of these statements to "I would have preferred not to have made a mistake" or "Perhaps XX doesn't like me, but YY might" or "I am shy most of the time but can enjoy being in a small group of people that I know well." These types of nuanced thoughts are not likely to come to mind automatically, but once you recognize the extremes, it's easier to shift them. Watch out for words that are laden with emotions. If you use more "boring" or neutral language, the words lose their sting.

WATCH OUT FOR LABELS

If you are in the habit of labeling yourself in negative ways in your thoughts, try saying such a thought out loud. What does the label mean? Is it accurate? Does it fit for all situations or just some? Would you label others in the same way for the same mistakes? Many people with social anxiety have a double standard that favors others over themselves. It's not fair to yourself to hold standards that are higher for you than for other people. Would you say these things to a person you cared about? That's you!

DON'T TRUST YOUR GUT

We are often told to "trust your gut" or "listen to your intuition." Yet you may be fooled if you follow this advice, as that is the root of what

EVIDENCE FOR AND AGAINST A THOUGHT

Thought: _____

_____

Evidence for	Evidence against

is called *emotional reasoning*—believing something to be true because it feels a certain way. The gut response of a person with social anxiety would probably be to back off, avoid, and not talk to new people because of fear. Your intuition might say the same thing—don't get involved, don't take a chance or a risk. An anxious person will almost always instinctively want to not be anxious, and not doing things will almost always bring relief. Try to see your gut reactions or intuition as just one piece of information. People who work to think realistically will try to make choices on the basis of multiple sources of information. Your gut may be one source of information, but also include your brain as well as the facts. You may be less prone to avoid social situations and improve over time.

LEARN TO THINK IN SHADES OF GRAY

It's easy to engage in all-or-none thinking. Ask yourself: Am I 100% convinced that these thoughts are accurate? How do I know that? These questions can help you think in shades of gray rather than black-and-white extremes. Most situations are not black and white, and it's helpful to assess things on a continuum from 0 to 100%. The gray zone is a bit boring but also more accurate most of the time.

EXAMINE PREDICTIONS ABOUT THE FUTURE

As you learned earlier in this chapter, biased thoughts may make negative predictions about the future. ("If I talk to Sonja, she will ignore me"; "If I speak out in class, others will think I'm stupid") These predictions can be enough to stop you from even taking the risk. But here are some questions you can ask yourself to deescalate the risk you see in a situation:

- What is the worst that could happen? How would I cope with that outcome?
- What is the best that could happen?
- What is the most likely thing that could happen?
- What is the probability that each of the above will happen?

It's important to ask the questions above in the order listed and end on the most likely option. While the worst-case scenario may be unlikely, the consequences could be dire.

Kevin is 20, single, and lonely. He thinks he's unappealing and boring. He'd like to ask a young woman he's tried to talk to a few times on a date. The worst-case scenario for Kevin may be that she says no and tells him she wouldn't go out with him even if she was desperate and lonely. He might then predict that he would never again have the nerve to try to date, as he would be so humiliated. The likelihood of this occurrence might be rated as low, but it would feel devastating if it happened. The best outcome would certainly be an enthusiastic yes, while the most likely would probably be "I'll check my calendar and get back to you in the morning." The most likely scenario as it plays out would probably be that the woman will chat with Kevin for a few minutes rather than walk away, and over the next few weeks their chats may become longer and they will eventually go out for coffee.

KEEP THE BIG PICTURE IN MIND

It's very easy to overestimate the importance of day-to-day events, so other helpful questions in any situation include:

- How much does this event matter to me right now?
- Will this matter a year from now, a month from now, a week from now?
- Have I ever been caught up in a worry only to have forgotten about it in a few days?

Amira came away from the doctor's appointment with her mother quite upset. On the way home from the doctor's appointment, Amira's mother suggested that they stop for lunch at a new restaurant that Amira wanted to try. Her mother offered to pay as a thank you to Amira for driving her. They had a nice lunch, and then Amira slept well that night, relieved that there was no pressure to take her mother anywhere for a few days. She realized that she tended to get frustrated after every appointment and that pattern had been occurring for some time. She appreciated that her mother acknowledged the effort that she put in—she hadn't been aware of that. She also resolved to think more about the overall patterns within the family and try to focus on what was important—her relationship with her brother and her own communication with others. She made a plan to sit down with her brother and discuss how to approach these issues in the future.

Learn to Be More Realistic and Develop Alternative Thoughts

After you've identified your automatic and anxiety-related thoughts, looked at them more realistically, and asked yourself some of the questions above, you will be ready to figure out some alternative thoughts. Often these thoughts are not radically different from the original but are kinder and gentler toward you. Think of it as softening your thoughts or sanding out their hard edges. Alternative thoughts have to be somewhat credible to be effective. For example, if you commonly see yourself as socially awkward and unskilled, you are not likely to believe a thought such as "I am suave and articulate." A more plausible alternative might be "I may say the wrong thing sometimes, but I'm trying my best" or "Many likable people are kind of awkward." Amira's thought "I am a doormat" could be realistically shifted to "I do not speak up for myself very often and then am resentful afterward."

> **PRACTICE EXERCISE 3: Adding alternative thoughts and consequences to self-monitoring**
>
> Consequences refer to what happened after the situation occurred. It is common to be anxious about "predicted consequences" such as someone might be upset or not like you. In the exercise, you can try predicting the consequences and then observe what actually happened. Were they different? Try this for yourself, using the form on page 111 (also available to download and print at *www.guilford.com/dobson3*-forms).

We learn best and most effectively by taking small steps, and this strategy is useful for adjusting our thinking as well. Try to shift your thoughts bit by bit rather than in big chunks. For example, the

ALTERNATIVE THOUGHTS AND CONSEQUENCES

Situation (date, time, event)	Automatic thought(s)	Feelings (include intensity, rating from 0–100)	Actions/behaviors	Alternative thoughts	Consequences

prediction "It will happen for sure, and it will be a catastrophe" can be shifted to "It has a high probability of happening and would be difficult to cope with" to "It might happen, and I have some ideas about what I would do if that is the case" to "I really have no idea." This scenario could be applied to a prediction regarding a relationship, a job, or a move across the country.

DO SOME RESEARCH TO FIGURE OUT OUTCOMES

There are in fact many times when an outcome can't be known. A useful strategy can be to try to figure it out by doing some research. I had a female client who was 30 and wanted to marry, have children, and grow old with another person. But she started predicting that she was becoming too old for anyone to be interested in starting a family with her, and was feeling sad and hopeless about the future. Most of her friends were not only married but pregnant, and she thought that her best option was to give up and adapt to spinsterhood. I suggested that she do some research to figure out whether her prediction was accurate. So she investigated the average age of marriage in different decades and in different countries around the world and discovered that the age of marriage had increased over the past 40 years and in many countries was now well over 30 years. After discussing her findings with me, she felt much more "average" and more hopeful.

While broad, population-level information could not directly help my client find a suitable partner, it shifted her thoughts and led to more hope and efforts to be involved with other people. She worked on completing an alternative thought chart, using opening an invitation to a baby shower as the situation. Her initial automatic thoughts were "I will never find a partner or have children" and "I'm too old and might as well give up." Her emotions were sadness (75/100), hopelessness (80/100), and some relief (25/100) at not having to try to date. Another thought was "I'll decline the invitation," but her action was to accept. After doing some research, her alternative thought was "I'm average, and most of my friends got married young." The consequences were reduced sadness but some trepidation at becoming more socially involved. A consequential thought was "I'll be open to trying."

Be Kind to Yourself: Self-Compassion

As noted earlier, holding a double standard is common among those with social anxiety. You may very well have much harsher thoughts about yourself than about others. You may give friends the benefit of the doubt or make excuses for them if they make mistakes, but not yourself. You may hold yourself to very high standards regarding your friendships, family, and work. These standards can get in the way and make it difficult to be kind to yourself or even try. A statement that has resonated with me is that "perfectionism is the enemy of the good." Being good enough is good enough!

> *Barry's friend Susan was frequently late to pick him up on the way to work, but Barry didn't raise the issue as he figured Susan had more important things to do than he had. As he hadn't raised it, Susan wasn't aware that he was concerned about it. Barry was worried that his boss noticed that he was frequently a few minutes late for work, whereas Susan was in a more senior position and so had more leeway with her schedule. When it was his turn to drive, Barry left early to make sure that he did not pick up Susan late. He was concerned about her waiting on the corner in the cold. This example typifies a double standard—Barry was more concerned about Susan's feelings than his own and was reluctant to raise any issues for fear of offending her. He was taking a risk with his boss, however, that was leading to anxiety for him.*

Self-compassion involves talking to yourself as you might to a dear friend. You are not likely to call them names or use accusatory language. It involves treating yourself kindly and speaking up for yourself as if you are as important as anyone else . . . because you are! It involves unconditional acceptance of who you are as a person; that does not mean you are not trying to make changes—we all are. We are all fallible human beings generally trying our best to live well.

Self-compassion is especially needed when your negative thoughts are accurate. People sometimes are treated badly, taken advantage of, bullied, or abused. When that is the case, the solution is to do something about the situation itself.

Amira made plans to talk to her brother about the lack of fairness in how they dealt with their mother's medical needs. He might not be willing to change his schedule to take her to appointments, but perhaps another solution could be found, such as asking another family member or friend to help out.

Moving Forward

Be kind to yourself. Talk to yourself and treat yourself as a good friend that you care a great deal about. Practice self-compassion and acceptance. We can fully accept ourselves as well as work on change. Now that you have an understanding of how to assess and shift your thoughts, you are in a better position to deal with the temptation of avoidance. Learning how to "avoid avoidance" is a crucial step in living well with social anxiety.

6

how to avoid the temptation of avoidance

It's natural to avoid situations, people, conversations, or anything else you find frightening. Avoidance brings quick relief and reduces discomfort, distress, and anxiety in the short term. But it maintains and worsens problems over the long term. It's a slippery slope. The short-term gain of relief from anxiety leads to the long-term pain of a constrained life. Think of a time that you put off making an important but difficult phone call—it likely became more and more difficult as time passed. Or a time when you declined an opportunity because of lack of confidence. That opportunity may not have come your way again. Through avoidance, life gradually becomes limited.

Jody has been thinking of signing up for a dating app. One of her new friends at work has encouraged her and offered to help pick out some photos and write her profile. Jody has kept telling her that she's too busy with work and wants to put it off until she has more time to focus on putting forth her best image. Jody is also thinking that she wants to wait until summer, once she has had a chance to update her wardrobe and take some flattering pictures. She can't afford to go shopping right now but is trying to save some money. She is very anxious about meeting new people and "putting herself out there" online for all to see.

Jesse, a server at a fast-food restaurant, knew that their boss wanted to arrange a meeting and was quite sure that they would be reprimanded or fired for being late several days in a row. They ducked into the washroom when the boss was around, avoided eye contact, and worked hard to seem busy. Nothing happened for several days, but Jesse's anxiety continued to escalate, and they called in sick on Friday. They did not have any shifts scheduled over the weekend and so felt relieved. They couldn't sleep on Sunday night, however, for fear that the boss would be in on Monday, and seriously considered calling in sick again.

Ryan was putting off working on his résumé. His mother kept leaving the half-finished printout on the kitchen table and repeatedly offered to help. He was sure he wouldn't get a job as he had no training or work experience. So what was the point? He didn't want to be rejected, although he did want to get his parents off his back. He sat down at the table and worked on the résumé for a few minutes, just enough to let his mother know that he had tried. He had little hope for change, so he went back into the basement to play video games.

Have you ever put something off? Made an excuse that you're too tired to go out, or have to leave an event early because you feel out of place? Sometimes we hope that problems will just magically disappear. All of us can plead guilty to procrastination and different types of avoidance for many different reasons. Procrastination is just one type of avoidance.

This chapter focuses on the biggest culprit that maintains and increases anxiety over time. Avoidance is very tempting and seductive as it provides immediate relief, which feels good when you're anxious. Avoidance can feel like a sensible choice. Has anyone ever said you'd feel better if you just relaxed or rested? Many people firmly believe that avoidance is a good thing. But psychological research strongly disputes that claim.

The Many Faces of Avoidance

Resisting the urge to avoid starts with understanding that there are common patterns to the ways people avoid social interactions due to anxiety.

Anxiety-Driven Choices about What to Do or Not Do

Some types of avoidance are obvious—you stay home, don't go out at all or answer your phone or text messages. Ryan goes out for long walks at night when other people are at home in bed. He may think "I'm getting some exercise," but he is avoiding contact with people. If you believe a friend is angry at you, you may ignore your friend's messages or walk the other way if you see them on the street. Avoiding leads to isolation. If you ignore requests to see people, invitations gradually stop coming. You don't resolve interpersonal problems.

Behavioral avoidance is the type of avoidance that typically comes to mind. Simply not doing something that is challenging is one form of behavioral avoidance; another is avoiding doing one activity by doing something else instead. This tactic provides a ready excuse, such as Jody's saying she is too busy to create an online profile for the dating app. It's easy to decline an invitation to go out by saying you have too much to do. There are many variations on "avoidance by substitution" of one activity for another. You might choose a job with lower pay and status to avoid taking on the responsibility of dealing with too many people. If you have to make decisions about other people, it may trigger socially anxious thoughts. I had a client who deliberately avoided managerial roles because he feared interpersonal conflict even though he would have been very good at these types of jobs.

Behavioral avoidance doesn't always mean not being present. You can avoid even when you're physically in a situation by looking down, sitting or standing alone, or trying to blend in by being quiet or appearing nondescript. This can involve trying to make sure that you don't wear unusual or revealing clothes, laugh too loud, or stand out from the group. It can involve sitting on the sidelines and working hard not to be noticed.

Avoidance in Conversations

Other types of avoidance are less obvious and can be quite subtle and tricky to figure out. There are many types of subtle avoidance. Have you ever avoided giving your opinion? Not taken a stand on a controversial topic? Deferred to others when asked what movie or restaurant you want to go to? All of these are common for people with social anxiety as the thought may be "I'll say the wrong thing" or "My preference doesn't count and probably will be seen as boring" or "Others won't like it." Are you overly agreeable even if you're not totally sure if you do agree? Fear of stating your opinion or disagreeing with others is a common type of avoidance during conversations.

Stating strong opinions can lead to disagreement and conflict. Conflict avoidance is familiar to many people and is common in social anxiety. Most of us do not want others to be irritated or angry at us. You may worry that you won't be able to express yourself well if you're upset, while the other person will remain able to do so. Have you ever thought of the best response after an argument is over? You may think your preferences or opinions are not as fully thought out or researched as others' might be. I learned many years ago that those who talk the most are often not the most well informed!

Emotional and Cognitive Avoidance

Do you avoid sharing personal information and think of yourself as a good listener? People who avoid sharing often worry about being judged and emotionally vulnerable so may ask questions rather than self-disclose. Trying to prevent uncomfortable feelings like anxiety, sadness, or vulnerability is emotional avoidance. Do you ever avoid going to see a sick person in the hospital so that you don't become sad? Or do you put off a difficult conversation because it is likely to trigger anxiety? Or go to a social function near the end of the scheduled time? If you start to experience tension or anxiety while in the situation, you can easily leave as quickly as possible. It's easy to avoid negative emotions by avoiding the situations that could trigger them.

Or maybe you avoid certain types of difficult thoughts or beliefs—cognitive avoidance. You might try to "just think positive or cheerful thoughts." You recognize that you're having anxiety-related thoughts and might purposely distract yourself in an attempt to feel better. Being distracted from and avoiding difficulties has a significant downside: You may not learn much about yourself. Also, by not thinking about the problems you're facing, you might actually delay or avoid solving the problems more directly.

Choosing Approach Instead of Avoidance

On the Monday of the week they were to meet with their boss, Jesse went shopping during their break, looking for a new video game that was advertised in a store nearby. It was expensive, but Jesse had already started planning how to spend the raise they would receive if they weren't fired. This is an example of cognitive avoidance. Instead, Jesse could have sat down in the back of the restaurant and prepared a list of positive comments they had heard from customers and a list of reasons for being viewed as a good employee, to present to the boss. They could have considered how best to begin the meeting and ways to manage the anxiety that could arise. This is an example of cognitive approach rather than avoidance.

Jesse's initial inclination was to avoid thinking about the upcoming meeting because it was anxiety provoking. It's easy to avoid thinking about something by scrolling through social media. Doing some planning ahead instead would be approaching rather than avoiding the situation. While planning would have required Jesse to experience some anxiety, it would also have led to problem solving. It's far more useful to approach than to avoid an anxiety-provoking thought, situation, or action.

Stop Trying to Feel Better

Escaping or avoiding something that is anxiety provoking brings relief and a quick reduction of anxiety. According to psychological theory and research, this reduction is very rewarding as people want to feel better and dislike being anxious. Another word used to describe reward is *reinforcement*—escape and avoidance are reinforced by the reduction of anxiety. Behaviors that are reinforced in this way tend to stick around. Think of a time when you wanted to approach a new person in a group. You walked toward the new person with a plan in your mind but became more and more nervous as you got closer. At the last second, the new person looked away, and you took the opportunity to go to the door and leave. You felt much less nervous and thought "I'll try again next time." It is likely to be more difficult the next time around as you did not make an attempt, learned nothing new, and did not build your confidence.

Repeated escape and avoidance have been shown to strongly maintain any anxious behavior over the long term. Avoidance leads to more avoidance. In fact, it is probably the single most important area to work on changing to live your best life with social anxiety. The graph below shows how avoidance quickly reduces anxiety in the moment.

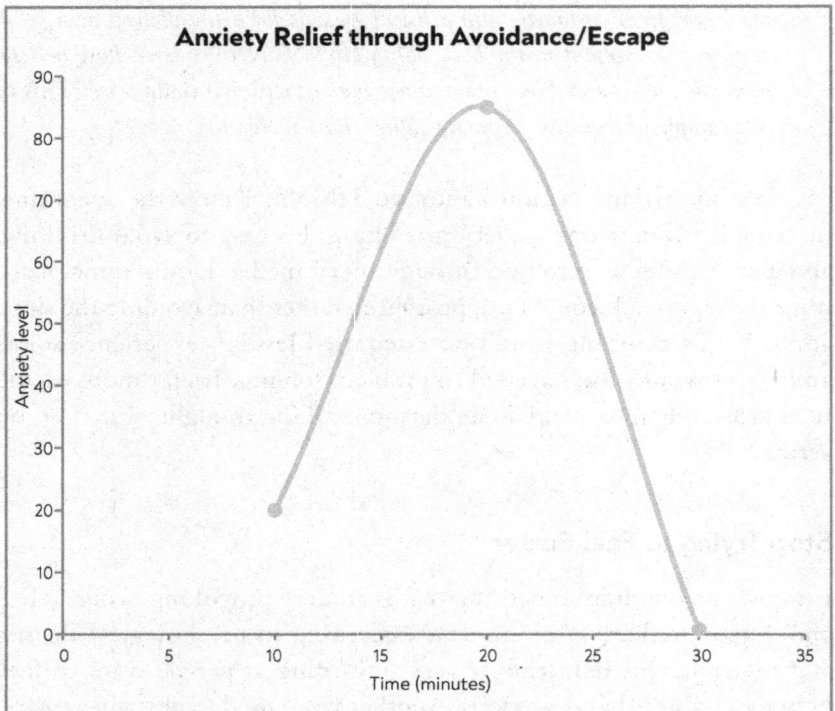

Anxiety Relief through Avoidance/Escape

When you leave a situation at the height of your anxiety, though, you only learn that avoidance is effective and not that your anxiety could have been reduced more effectively and enduringly with time or other strategies.

Avoidance has numerous consequences—as noted above, people who avoid do not learn anything new other than perhaps that they can't (or choose not to) do something. Other negative consequences of avoidance are limited opportunities, lack of information to dispute thoughts, a restricted life, and worsening problems over time. Some people with chronic social anxiety disorder do not actually experience high levels of anxiety because they are very successful avoiders and seldom challenge themselves. They do not allow themselves to experience distress. People who avoid may not feel much anxiety but may have a host of other feelings such as loneliness, sadness, guilt, and frustration.

Build Confidence through Discomfort

Avoidance leads to an erosion of self-esteem and confidence whereas trying new things tends to build confidence even when they don't work out as hoped or expected. As Eleanor Roosevelt said, "Do one thing every day that scares you." You will become less scared over time. I have often said to anxious clients that the best way to build self-esteem is to do "hard stuff." Once we have taken some action, it is no longer possible to say that we can't! Even if we have tried something that did not work out as we hoped, we put in some effort, have learned something, and are more likely to try something again.

As noted in Chapter 5, at times societal or cultural beliefs promote the idea that we are doing the right thing through avoidance. We may hear directives such as "Avoid or reduce your stress," "Avoid any triggers that could make you uncomfortable," or "When you're feeling stressed, stay home and take it easy." I have a colleague who makes the statement "No one ever got better from a psychological problem by staying home and going to bed." Our fears tend to increase when we have lots of time to think about how bad things are. Our estimate of our ability to cope with the fears tends to decrease. People who say these things have good intentions and are trying to be reassuring. However, avoiding things that are anxiety provoking does nothing to bolster our ability to cope with them or reduce our fears. So temporary relief from anxiety truly is a problem and creates more problems over time.

Much of the time it's difficult to estimate risks. People who are prone to anxiety tend to overestimate risks. Risks certainly do exist, however. While some things are clearly dangerous and a "threat to life and limb," most situations require a judgment call that will vary from person to person. While it is possible to calculate the risks of dying in a plane crash or motor vehicle accident, it is very difficult, if not impossible, to figure out social risks. If a situation is objectively risky, it is sensible to avoid it. Very few social situations are objectively risky, but going to a nightclub along a dark alley and walking home alone would be foolish. If a situation is humiliating or shame-producing, it might be wise to avoid it as well. These situations include any physical, sexual, psychological, or emotional abuse. Typically, a person is going to weigh the pros and cons of approach and avoidance. If you are afraid of flying but have an opportunity for a fabulous, free Caribbean vacation, you might consider getting on an airplane. Some people would, and some would not. Later in this chapter, you'll learn about strategic avoidance.

Reduce Avoidance through Repeated Practice

Becoming proficient and confident in a new skill usually requires repeated practice. This applies to learning a new language, swimming, playing an instrument, and learning social skills as well as learning how to reduce anxiety. You may have heard the term *exposure therapy*—it's commonly used when learning about mental health treatments for anxiety. I have had prospective clients ask "Are you going to make me do _____?" (insert the word for whatever you might be afraid of). I hear trepidation in their voice, which is perfectly understandable. When asked this question, I always say no. It's crucial for you to choose what you do or don't do. A great deal of scientific research has shown, however, that exposure therapy is the single most beneficial intervention for all anxiety disorders. We know from research findings that it's important to confront what you're afraid of and gradually challenge yourself in a systematic way to face your fears.

Exposure: You Can Confront Your Fears

We just reviewed how exposure therapy works for social anxiety: You (1) choose to stop trying to feel better, which (2) frees you to notice you can tolerate some discomfort, and (3) gain the confidence to keep practicing. Essentially exposure involves counteracting natural avoidance. You prove to yourself that you can handle situations that cause you anxiety, and your body also gradually learns to become more comfortable.

Most people with social anxiety disorder tend to avoid many different aspects of social functioning, which only reinforces their continued use of avoidance. If you're wondering how exposure therapy differs from forcing yourself to go to work or attend family functions, which doesn't seem to improve your social anxiety, it's the gradual and systematic nature of planned exposure that matters.

Taking risks is extremely important to your wellness, but they must be calculated risks—that's what we mean by *systematic* and *gradual*. To have benefit, exposure should lead you to experience some but not excessive levels of anxiety. Too little anxiety won't be enough to put you in your discomfort zone so you can prove your fears wrong. Too much anxiety can make it difficult to pay attention to what is going on in the situation. In the extreme you might even panic and escape, which just reinforces the anxiety you had to begin with and may discourage you from trying the same thing again. As you become more comfortable with the situation, you can move on to the next step.

> Exposure should be structured, planned,
> and predictable. It must be within your control.

The Importance of Planning and Structure

People sometimes ask, "If exposure to others helps people recover from social anxiety, why am I still anxious? I'm around people every day. Shouldn't this have worked by now?" Natural exposure—like being in a classroom full of students day after day—may not be sufficient or helpful for several reasons. Some naturally occurring exposure is unpredictable and does not feel in your control. If you are suddenly called on to speak in class, you may blurt something out but not feel very good about it. Or you might find yourself in a crowded supermarket even though you chose to shop at a time of day when the store is usually empty. Both examples involve unexpected and unplanned incidents. You likely avoid certain types of encounters (like being in a crowded store) or dread them (being called on in class). These encounters may be brief or negative. Brief encounters tend not to be long enough to give you much time to respond, and if they catch you off guard, you may be more likely to interpret them negatively. While they are occurring, you may instinctively engage in negative thoughts or self-focused behaviors (such as tuning out and focusing only on how anxious you are) or try to create "safety" within the situation, such as avoiding being the center of attention, rather than responding in a more analytical way as you might in a more predictable situation.

Identifying Your Safety Behaviors

Psychologists sometimes use the term *safety behaviors* to describe the tricky and subtle types of avoidance discussed earlier in this chapter. Safety behaviors are one of the main reasons natural recovery from social anxiety may not occur or tends to be slow. These behaviors (or thoughts) reduce anxiety, so they are reinforcing and will continue. Exposure will help only if you experience some anxiety. In fact, in the context of exposure therapy the term *exposure* means *exposure to anxiety and discomfort* rather than to the situation itself!

The Social Coping Scale on pages 125–126 shows different possible safety behaviors. Many of the items on this scale are things you probably believe to be helpful but actually minimize the effectiveness of actions that you take and prevent you from learning how to reduce your social anxiety. For example, distraction could mean that you're focusing on something positive while anxious. Distraction includes daydreaming, tuning out, or deliberately thinking of something else. These are all types of internal avoidance. Distraction takes you out of the situation mentally, making you less likely to notice what is going on. You might miss cues that other people are providing and get mixed

SOCIAL COPING SCALE

For each item, circle or highlight the number that would appropriately reflect your own experience.

1 = Rarely occurs
2 = Occasionally occurs
3 = Occurs about half the time
4 = Frequently occurs
5 = Occurs almost all the time

1. I go only to social events where I know what to expect.   1   2   3   4   5

2. I tend to steer the conversation toward the other person.   1   2   3   4   5

3. I keep my hands and arms tense or clench my hands to prevent them from shaking during social events.   1   2   3   4   5

4. I try to act aloof or indifferent to what others may think of me.   1   2   3   4   5

5. I have a drink to calm down before I go out.   1   2   3   4   5

6. I avoid eye contact and may even wear dark sunglasses.   1   2   3   4   5

7. I only go out with someone who is quite self-confident.   1   2   3   4   5

8. I tend to worry about how I will manage during an upcoming social event.   1   2   3   4   5

9. I avoid sharing personal information about myself with others.   1   2   3   4   5

10. I tend to be overly apologetic.   1   2   3   4   5

11. I take an anti-anxiety medication (e.g., Ativan) before I go out.   1   2   3   4   5

12. I tend to be the one who helps out with the drinks, food, or clean-up at social functions.   1   2   3   4   5

13. I avoid shaking people's hands because my palms are sweaty.   1   2   3   4   5

14. I try to blend in.   1   2   3   4   5

15. I think of myself as a better listener than conversationalist.   1   2   3   4   5

16. Before I go out, I rehearse what I will do or say in detail.   1   2   3   4   5

(continued)

1 = Rarely occurs
2 = Occasionally occurs
3 = Occurs about half the time
4 = Frequently occurs
5 = Occurs almost all the time

17. I only go to those social events where I know most of the people.   1 2 3 4 5

18. I tend to be agreeable.   1 2 3 4 5

19. I worry about the impression I'm making on others.   1 2 3 4 5

20. I am prone to daydreaming, fantasizing, or "tuning out."   1 2 3 4 5

21. I tend to leave social events fairly early, as soon as I notice other people starting to leave.   1 2 3 4 5

22. While others are speaking, I try to think of the next question to ask or comment to make.   1 2 3 4 5

23. I avoid going out if I am feeling anxious.   1 2 3 4 5

24. I tend to worry about how I came across following a social event.   1 2 3 4 5

25. I tend to drink too much when I'm out socially.   1 2 3 4 5

26. I focus on how I feel physically when I'm out socially.   1 2 3 4 5

27. During a social event, I focus on how I think I'm coming across to others and sometimes miss what was said.   1 2 3 4 5

28. I tend to talk less than others.   1 2 3 4 5

29. Once a social event is over, I spend a lot of time going over it and analyzing what I said and did.   1 2 3 4 5

30. I try my best to "get through" the social event with the least possible anxiety.   1 2 3 4 5

31. I focus on controlling my own breathing during a social event.   1 2 3 4 5

32. I dress in an inconspicuous manner to avoid being the center of attention.   1 2 3 4 5

33. I focus on trying to relax during a social event.   1 2 3 4 5

34. I use disclaimers when I state an opinion; for example "I could be wrong, but . . ." or "I probably don't know what I'm talkingabout, but. . . ."

35. I prefer to socialize outside my own home.   1 2 3 4 5

up in the conversation. The same thing happens if you avoid eye contact. If you wear sunglasses, not only will you avoid eye contact, but others will probably not approach you to talk. The same "stay away" messages can be sent if you wear a ball cap or hoodie, like Ryan. You may be in a social situation, but if you are at the same time avoiding eye contact, standing in a corner not talking to others, or looking for an opportunity to leave at the earliest appropriate time, you are not fully engaged—instead you are working hard to minimize anxiety, and consequently not fully exposing yourself to the anxiety or the situation.

PRACTICE EXERCISE 1: Social Coping Scale

Fill out the Social Coping Scale on pages 125–126 (also available to download and print at *www.guilford.com/dobson3-forms*), which is designed to assess people's reactions to social situations. Social situations or events involve interactions between two or more individuals. They can occur at school, work, or in almost any place and may involve people you know or don't know. The items in the list can apply before, during, or following a social event. Some of these will involve "easy outs." Identifying these easy outs can eventually help you reduce their use.

What patterns do you notice in your completed questionnaire? Do the thoughts and actions you ranked as occurring fairly frequently actually help you or do they interfere with your functioning? Which ones tend to be temporary "crutches" and which are "easy outs," which help you remain anxious rather than help build your confidence? What would be one behavior that you could drop?

Jody was pleased that she was invited to a potluck dinner over the Thanksgiving holiday. She was excited to go and had been worried that she would be homesick for her family as they lived far away and she couldn't afford to travel home. She decided to make a casserole for the event and arrived right at the designated time. She was surprised that very few people were there yet, and she offered to help out in the kitchen. A few women were quite busy getting things ready and gave her a job cutting up vegetables. She was relieved to have a task to do that didn't involve talking. She stayed in the kitchen and on the sidelines for much of the time as people started to arrive and get their plates of food. After she ate quickly, she noticed that some of the children and teenagers were heading into the basement, and she went down as well, spending the remainder of the evening playing games and watching the children.

While Jody went to the potluck, she engaged in several safety behaviors, like staying in the kitchen, helping with the preparations and serving, and going into the basement after the meal. All of these actions limited her interactions with other adults. While it was positive that she attended, she managed her anxiety with the use of these actions. When she attends the next social function, she could consider pushing herself to talk to some of the adults and be "less helpful" in the kitchen.

ASK YOURSELF THE RIGHT QUESTIONS

We all avoid. What is important in this context is what and how we avoid related to anxiety. Some avoidance is obvious; some is subtle. It's important to ask yourself honest questions and spend some time thinking about what you do. People with social phobia are often masters of excuses. Do you make excuses to avoid parties and other contact? As described earlier, safety behaviors including distracting yourself (internal avoidance) keep your anxiety low in the short term but alive and well in the long term because they reinforce themselves rather than your capacity to expose yourself to social situations without unbearable anxiety. They will make exposure less effective and progress toward reduced anxiety slower. What did you learn about your avoidance and coping behaviors from completing the Social Coping Scale?

USE SAFETY BEHAVIORS AS CRUTCHES, NOT EASY OUTS

Yes, identifying your safety behaviors is intended to reduce your reliance on avoidance. But it's important to be kind to yourself as well as realistic. Be aware of excuses and safety behaviors but also use your judgment. Plan to use a "crutch" if you really need it. A crutch is anything that can help you feel in control of the process, so that you feel better able to face an anxiety-provoking situation. Just as physical crutches allow an injury to heal by reducing stress on a fracture, a psychological crutch can help give you enough courage that you will no longer need the help. The crutch helps you get into the situation rather than continuing to avoid it. Compare an easy out to a crutch: Easy outs help you avoid the situation, while crutches help you get in. See the box below for examples.

You may want to experiment with some psychological crutches to see what it feels like to use them. Use your crutch only when planned and necessary, and don't use it to escape the discomfort of social anxiety altogether. If you do need to avoid an anxiety-provoking situation, make sure you place yourself back in it as soon as possible to complete the task. The longer you wait to return, the more difficult it will be.

Taking One Step at a Time

It would be exhausting and unhelpful to work on reducing your anxiety all the time. Remember your goals and values and carefully choose what to focus on. Practicing exposure can take time, and the change that occurs is slower and more gradual than the anxiety relief that comes with avoidance. The graph on page 130 describes the pattern for exposure.

Examples of Easy Outs versus Crutches

✗ Easy out: Have your friend order your dinner at the restaurant.

✓ Crutch: Tell yourself that if you are not ready to speak when the waiter comes, you will simply say you need a few more minutes to look at the menu.

✗ Easy out: Take the stairs so you don't have to stand in the elevator with other people.

✓ Crutch: Remind yourself that if you become very anxious when you are in the elevator you can get off at the next floor and take a break before getting back on.

✗ Easy out: Avoid going to a party that you're invited to and say that you'll go "next time."

✓ Crutch: Go to the party, but plan to leave at a specific time. If needed, take a break in the washroom.

Anxiety Reduction through Exposure

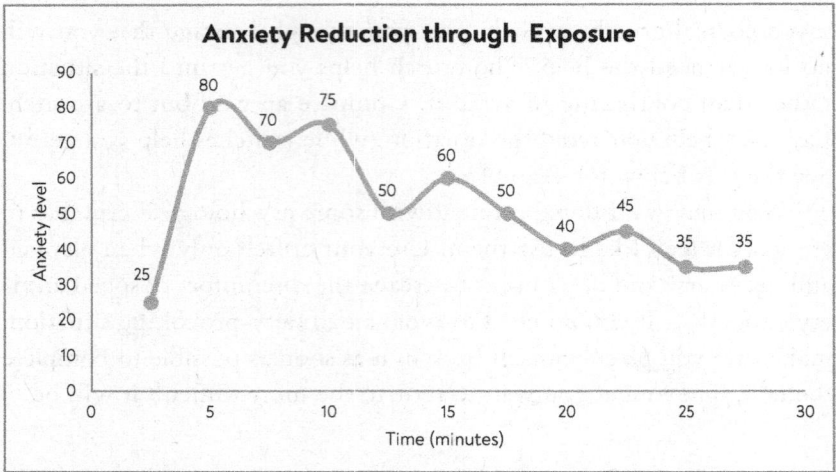

Remember as well that even if your anxiety decreases slowly, you will learn many other things from facing it. You'll learn to tolerate anxiety and that it will not hurt you. You'll learn that you are capable of trying something new. Many people learn that the situation they have feared and avoided for years is not that scary at all! You may learn something about others if you are fully engaged in the situation and not distracted. You probably will feel more positive about yourself and gradually develop confidence.

Assessing Your Progress

Which of the following characterize your use of exposure?

❑ You're doing it gradually, tackling easier, more manageable steps first and more challenging steps later.

❑ It is deliberate and planned.

❑ You're doing it in the actual anxiety-provoking situation or its closest approximation.

❑ You're doing it in a variety of settings or with a variety of people.

❑ It causes your anxiety to rise to a moderate (not extreme or unmanageable) level—expect to feel uncomfortable.

❑ You planned for a "crutch" (a way to help you feel more control, such as a "time out") that can be used if needed.

❑ You do it often.

❑ You do it for more than a few minutes at a time.

❑ It is planned according to your goals and consistent with your values.

❑ You're aware that you use subtle avoidance strategies during the exposure (such as distraction, alcohol, leaving early, avoiding eye contact) and you are trying to gradually minimize them.

❑ You record it to monitor progress, perhaps on your phone or calendar.

> *After a sleepless night Monday, Jesse went to work at the restaurant bright and early Tuesday morning and, fed up with being anxious and avoiding their boss, made an appointment to meet with the boss at 10:00 A.M. Jesse knew they had a pattern of avoiding eye contact, rushing through questions and comments to leave meetings early, and being overly agreeable. They decided to think of things that made them a good employee and the positive comments they had gotten from customers, and give a list of these to their boss. The boss looked a bit surprised by Jesse's request for a 10:00 A.M. meeting but agreed to it. Jesse was pleased to have "taken the bull by the horns" rather than skulked around all day trying to avoid attention. During the meeting, the boss did comment on the late work arrivals but acknowledged that Jesse generally worked hard and was a good employee. He asked Jesse to do their best to be on time and said that some pay would be docked if the lateness continued. At the end of the meeting, there was no indication that Jesse would lose their job. In fact being fired seemed unlikely given the shortage of workers. Jesse was very pleased with the meeting and thanked the boss for agreeing to it.*

This situation was very difficult and anxiety provoking for Jesse. It might not seem like exposure therapy, but it certainly exposed Jesse to anxiety, and it was consistent with their goals and values as work was important to Jesse and they very much wanted to keep their job. Jesse planned it in advance, and the request to meet was within their control. Think of how much more anxiety provoking it would have been to wait for the boss to request the meeting. Jesse would have continued to be highly anxious, with thoughts disrupting their sleep and even worsening their lateness.

> *Jody was in the lunchroom at work one day. She tended to have her lunch early to get some peace and quiet and solitude. She was leafing through a magazine when she heard someone open the fridge behind her. She did not turn around, but the person took something out and came around and sat down at the next table. It was a new employee that she had heard about but had not yet met. She nodded and smiled at him. He smiled back but appeared somewhat shy. She recognized a fellow shy person and decided that she would try to make him feel welcome. She introduced herself and said she had been with the company for only about six months, so if he had any questions about what the orientation had been like, she would be happy to talk to him. He responded by introducing himself as well and said that he had just moved to the city. In the conversation that followed, Jody was able to recommend some local resources that she had recently discovered.*

Jody's perception that the new employee was shy allowed her kindness to overcome her social anxiety, so it felt easier than usual to initiate a conversation. It is much more difficult to approach someone who is perceived as sophisticated, highly skilled, or in a different social category. Imagine for a moment that you were suddenly required to have a conversation with a celebrity that you've admired for years or a renowned international leader. Most of us would be at a loss for words! Jody could plan to ask her new coworker about the resources she had recommended the next time she saw him. A next step could be starting a conversation with another colleague in the lunchroom to add a bit more challenge.

Strategies for Embracing Exposure Practice

Exposure practice works well when you make it deliberate. It helps if you can incorporate a sense of fun and even adventure.

What to Try for Different Fears

Use your imagination to figure out what you could try out—here are some ideas to consider.

1. **If you are afraid of public speaking,** speak up in meetings at work, go to a public lecture and ask questions, offer to make a toast at a wedding, take a drama class, tell a joke at a family gathering. Perhaps the most difficult of these exposure ideas would be signing up for an improvisation comedy workshop! In the city where I live, there was a mental health comedy troupe that did improv training that culminated in an evening production. A difficult but fun course!

2. **If you struggle to make small talk,** say hello and then later on speak to strangers on elevators, in waiting rooms, and in lines, talk to cashiers in stores, give compliments, talk to neighbors on the street, express an everyday and then a controversial opinion. Interest in the weather is something everyone has in common.

3. **If you dislike being the center of attention,** take an aerobics or Zumba class, say something incorrect on purpose, spill your drink, drop something, ask for help in a store, talk about yourself, wear a T-shirt inside out, deliberately slur your words. These ideas may seem odd, but they can be approached in the spirit of fun. I had a client who was practicing spilling her drinks so often that her friends became more embarrassed than she did!

4. **If you're afraid to eat or drink in front of others,** do not eat a snack at your desk, but go to the lunchroom at work or school, eat alone in a food court, invite people over for coffee or a meal. It's often easier to eat foods like sandwiches and more difficult to eat "sloppy" foods like spaghetti and meatballs. If this applies to you, start with foods that seem less potentially messy and work toward messier ones.

5. **If you're afraid of job interviews,** apply for many jobs (even jobs you aren't interested in), practice interviews with family or friends, arrange informational interviews. Role-play interviews; switching spots with someone else allows you to see things from different points of view.

6. **If you're anxious around strangers,** go to a mall or super-market, walk down a busy street, read alone in a library, make eye contact with someone while riding a bus or train. Sit down next to someone on the subway and acknowledge them by nodding your head. If they don't respond, don't take it personally—they might just be surprised. Try it with different people for practice. On the other hand, sometimes it's wise to be cautious; see the box below.

What other ways can you think of that will help you practice exposure?

When to Plan Deliberate Avoidance

It's important to remember that it's not wise to approach all feared situations. When planning exposure involving initiating interactions with strangers, for example, you obviously must exercise commonsense caution. Planned avoidance can be strategic. Strategic avoidance means that it is deliberate and planful. If you decide the risks of taking an action outweigh the potential benefits, you may decide to avoid it. For instance, people stay in jobs or relationships that have problems but have benefits as well. Sometimes the anticipated anxiety of an activity may be so great that you decide to start with a related but easier activity. At times, you may try doing something and realize that the anxiety is much greater than you anticipated; if so, deliberately scale it back. I had a client who kept persisting despite intense physical anxiety to the point of vomiting—persisting in this way only made it worse.

The key is to be aware of your temptation to use avoidance, give it some serious consideration, and persist with change. This does not mean throwing common sense to the wind. Be aware, be kind to yourself, and try new things in gradual but consistent ways. Persistence over time will help a great deal, but we all decide that some activities or situations are not the best exposure practices for us.

How to Keep Practice Going over Time

1. **Encourage courage!** Exposure takes courage, so always give yourself credit for trying something new. People tend to regret things that they didn't do rather than what they did do.

2. **Random acts of exposure.** You may have heard of the Random Acts of Kindness Foundation, which encourages people to engage in small daily activities to be kind to others. As a person with social anxiety, you should practice random acts of exposure. I have shifted the phrase to encourage you to engage in small daily exposure activities. Small and frequent acts go a long way over time.

3. **Mindful exposure.** While you practice random acts of exposure, try to be fully aware of what you are doing and focus completely on the present moment. Being fully mindful means avoiding distraction, being aware of but not trying to shift how you feel and think. We can learn a great deal, and being mindful creates some "space" and generally helps us accept what is happening and get a little less caught up in it.

Being a Good Observer

Earlier in this book I stressed the idea that social anxiety weakens our powers of observation. We divert our attention by filtering what we see and hear through a self-referential lens. We also focus on internal sensations and thoughts related to our anxiety and not on what is happening around us. Since we have only a finite amount of attention, focusing much of it internally leaves little for concentrating on what is going on around us. Consequently, we may miss many parts of conversations, social cues, or nonverbal communication. Here are some exercises to help you develop your observational muscle.

PRACTICE EXERCISE 2: Go to a local park, sit on a bench, and be observant

Play an observation game with yourself—count how many people walk by who are wearing hats or glasses over 20 minutes. Invent stories about families that you see playing nearby or a couple that walks by. Are they having an argument or planning a vacation? Are they brother and sister or in a different type of relationship? Look for possible clues.

PRACTICE EXERCISE 3: Go to the park the next day and walk on the path rather than sit on the bench

Look directly at every person that you walk by rather than at the path or in the distance. Nod, smile, or say hello. Notice the responses that you get. Some might be surprised or not notice whereas others may seem friendly.

PRACTICE EXERCISE 4: Walk down a busy street looking down at the sidewalk

Be aware of your thoughts and feelings—you will not have any information about the people who walk by other than perhaps what shoes they are wearing. Thoughts may pop into your mind, such as "They are looking at me and thinking that I'm weird." You may feel self-conscious.

PRACTICE EXERCISE 5: Try this experiment again but looking around you and at the people who walk by

Observe carefully. Notice the difference between what you think and what you do. It's an exercise in turning from an inner to an outer focus.

PRACTICE EXERCISE 6: Be a little nosy

There are many ways to be observant, depending on where you are and what the situation is. Try the following:

- Listen to conversations when you are on public transit—what do people talk about?
- Look into other people's grocery carts when you go to the supermarket—what do you think they might be planning to make for dinner? How many people are in the household?
- If you are with someone else, make up games or stories about your environment. I used to do this when my children were young—when you see someone walking by, think about what their life might be like. Where are they going? What have they been doing today?

You may have an automatic thought that these strategies are somewhat nosy, but all of these situations are in public rather than private spaces.

Observational and listening skills require you to be present in the situation rather than have your mind somewhere else. They also limit the use of subtle avoidance strategies such as avoiding looking at people. In effect, they take you out of yourself and into your environment. The goal is to move from self-focused attention to an external focus on the people in your environment and the environment you are living in.

Living Well through Reducing Avoidance

Avoidance maintains fear. There are many types of avoidance—some obvious and some very subtle, such as avoiding eye contact or tuning out during a conversation. In this chapter, we have discussed many different ways that people with social anxiety avoid challenging themselves, which gives their problems "fuel" to grow and thrive. Many people believe that avoidance is helpful, but it is not unless it is deliberate and planned. Exposure to situations that make you anxious is the most effective strategy available to counteract avoidance. This chapter presented many different strategies and methods to use exposure. To help reduce anxiety and decrease avoidance, exposure should be gradual, continue until anxiety is reduced (even a bit), and be frequent. It should be done with awareness, and it helps to be fully engaged in the situation.

Strategies to try to include:

1. **Gradual practice**—do something easy to start with and work toward something a bit more difficult. Try to do something anxiety provoking every day—persist with practice.

2. **Practice with awareness** of your thoughts and reactions. You may surprise yourself, when something that you expected to be difficult turns out not to be. At times, situations may be more difficult than you expect, or something unpredictable might happen. It is important in these cases not to bow out and avoid situations at the height of your anxiety—instead scale back your exposure and try something somewhat easier.

3. **Practice random acts of exposure.** Take opportunities as they come up. Make a game of it when you can—many ideas were presented for practicing observation skills and directing your focus externally rather than internally. Practice requires courage—give yourself lots of credit for all that you try.

Moving Forward

Now that you have learned strategies to practice doing what you fear and have more confidence in your abilities to manage your anxiety and your thoughts, we will turn to ways to develop skills for everyday life. These involve communicating with other people in many different ways and situations.

PART THREE

living your best life

7

how to make the connections you want

Ryan felt isolated and different from other people. He was beginning to realize that others tended to give him a wide berth in response to his appearing standoffish and distant. He had recently joined an in-person gaming group and was planning to attend a meeting but was very nervous about his discomfort with basic interactions, like introducing himself and starting conversations. Usually he avoided others and waited for them to approach him, but they seldom did. So he faded into the background or appeared disagreeable. He was not feeling optimistic about the meeting but was determined to go.

After six months at her new job, Jody felt work was going quite well. She had put in many hours and taken on projects with three colleagues, who had invited her out to lunch to discuss work with them a few times. But she didn't feel comfortable inviting them or other coworkers to do anything non-work-related and she hadn't made any new friends outside of work. Bored and lonely, Jody was beginning to dread the weekends and found that even the evenings were draggy and long. She missed her family and felt very alone.

Just like Ryan and Jody, you are probably uncomfortable with trying to make friends and may lack confidence in your skills for meeting people in different settings. This chapter offers some strategies for improving and practicing social skills to live your best life. With practice comes confidence and more opportunities to meet people. It's also important to challenge your worries about your social skills and thoughts about inadequacy. Having "good enough" social skills is good enough!

What Makes It Difficult to Reach Out?

Like Ryan and Jody, you might avoid reaching out to people for several reasons—anxiety, self-doubt, lack of skills and practice, as well as infrequent opportunity. Beliefs can also hold you back. If you avoid the initial phases of relationships, it's difficult to meet people and figure out who you might have things in common with. Reaching out lets others know you're interested in them and often feels scary as others may say no and reject you. It's easier to wait until you're approached, and yet that may take a long time or may not happen at all. You may worry that you don't know how to form relationships. Self-doubt leads to avoidance. So you put things off and feel isolated and incapable.

You might not know whether you lack social skills or are just too anxious to try out the skills you do have. The good news is that it doesn't really matter. Whether you lack skills or are not confident in the skills that you do have, it's important to learn about and practice different types of skills. If you think you have good skills but are anxious about trying them out, practice leads to increased confidence and reduced anxiety. Gradual practice improves skills and confidence, provides exposure therapy, and increases social connections, so is a plus in all ways. Both learning and practicing provide opportunity. Opportunity is a way to minimize avoidance with the positive side effect of making friends. The main "risk" is that you might improve and have a richer life. Of course, you will be anxious along the way, but since you already are, you have nothing to lose.

Social skills require direct practice and immersion in situations. Could you learn to swim by reading a book about it, or would you need to get into the pool? Most of us learn to dog-paddle before we try an elegant dive, and many never become expert at or even attempt the dive. The important thing is to get out there and try things out. No one can make connections with others by not being around others! Unfortunately, many of us avoid trying for fear of failure—a key attitude in social anxiety.

> **Practice provides opportunity.**

Strong Social Connections Improve Your Health

Is the anxiety worth it? Yes! People are social beings. You want to have more connections with others and improve the relationships that you do have. People who are socially anxious feel lonely and isolated. Social connections and feeling like you are part of a community are good predictors of both your physical and mental health. Isolation contributes to depression as well as other health conditions. When you're isolated and no one sees you, it's easy to slip into bad habits related to eating, sleeping, and exercise. It's easy to drink too much when no one is around or to have little structure to your days.

Many people who are socially anxious say they find "chitchat," small talk, and "networking" to be superficial activities. It's understandable to prefer to have deeper and more meaningful conversations. Yet it's impossible to go from not knowing someone at all to instant personal connection. Small talk is a way to meet people, to get to know them to see if you have things in common and are compatible. Hopefully, small talk leads to big talk! It's easy to avoid and dismiss the initial parts of conversations. It's also a "push–pull" type of feeling—simultaneously wanting something and being scared to try it. However, having more people in your life will reduce isolation *and* improve your health.

What Exactly Are Social Skills?

Social skills and communication skills are the same thing. We learn to communicate from the time shortly after we are born, when we lock eyes with our caregiver, to when we learn to speak. We continue to learn throughout our lives. Without communication, we could not get our needs met. Communication is a complex process and involves facial expression, body language, what we say, and how we say it. It's the tone and volume of our voice. In our world, it can be in-person, on the telephone, via email, text, or video. It can be direct or indirect. We communicate when we are talking as well as when we are not talking—with our words as well as our silences.

The good news is that there is no magic in social skills—they are learned like any other skills. There are no absolutes in terms of what are considered good social skills. The most important thing is to be open to experimentation and observation. At times you'll have to use trial and error to see what works. This requires observing what happens and having the courage to try again.

While it may sound frustrating, there are many different things to keep in mind about learning and using social skills. What may work well for an older professional at a conference may not work well at all for a young adult in a club. What might work for Jody might not work well for Ryan. For example, a woman inviting another woman out for lunch would be likely to use different words or suggest different locations than a young man initiating a conversation about video games. While I may be uncomfortable with the use of "foul" language, not using it may be seen as prudish in certain situations. I may recommend having open body language with direct eye contact, which could be seen as aggressive in some cultures where deference is valued. While you need to keep many considerations in mind, you'll encounter lots of individual differences as well. Learn to be a good observer.

> Be open
> to experimenting and observing.

PRACTICE EXERCISE 1: The interview

Think of a person who is highly socially skilled—perhaps one who is suave, articulate, and an excellent public speaker. Others admire this person and aspire to that level of skillfulness. Perhaps it's someone you know or a public figure, such as a politician, musician, or actor. Take a few moments to consider what skills they have that you respect—perhaps it's openness, the ability to convince others, or something about their facial expressions. Perhaps they come across with enthusiasm, friendliness, or passion. Sometimes we use the word *charismatic* to describe these characteristics, and others may be attracted to such people like flies. It can be hard to put a finger on these skills, but consider them carefully.

Now imagine that your task is to interview this person for a research paper. You are required to write their profile and include lots of information. What are your automatic thoughts? How do you feel? How will you approach this interview? Are you tempted to ask someone else to take over?

Most of us would feel intimidated if we were called on to interview or even talk to the most socially skilled person we can think of. Barack Obama is generally thought of as being a gifted public speaker. If you were attending an event where he showed up, would you approach him or walk the other way? Many people worry about making mistakes when faced with famous people, such as accidentally stepping on their toe, shaking their hand incorrectly, tripping, or saying exactly the wrong thing. I had a socially gifted student who was leading a practice group with me for people with social anxiety. He demonstrated a skill with such aplomb that when he asked for volunteers to try it out no one volunteered. They feared that they would not measure up. They all looked at the floor and hoped that someone else would have the courage to try!

PRACTICE EXERCISE 2: The interview revisited

Think of a specific person you've met and would like to get to know better. This person comes across as likable and friendly but is far from the most socially skilled person you can think of. Sometimes they may say silly things, laugh at inappropriate times, or accidentally interrupt others. They make mistakes once in a while. And yet they seem to have lots of friends, and others enjoy being around them. What qualities do they have that make them seem approachable and friendly?

Now imagine your task is to interview this second person for a research paper. You're required to write their profile and include lots of information. What are your automatic thoughts? How do you feel? How will you approach this interview? Are you tempted to ask someone else to take over?

Notice which of the two people in Exercises 1 and 2 you would be drawn to speak to. While a famous person might be very interesting to talk to, a person who makes mistakes at times comes across as human and approachable. It helps most of us feel better about our own gaffes as well and equalizes the relationship. Such people tend to be easier to talk to and even make us feel good about ourselves.

Making Mistakes and Challenging Perfectionism

Many anxious people struggle with perfectionism and hold themselves to very high social standards. They judge themselves harshly and hesitate to try new things for fear of making mistakes. They put things off. But anyone learning new skills makes mistakes—it's how we learn. People who are socially anxious apply these standards to their social "performance." Worrying about not being "good enough" and about making social gaffes is a real deterrent to trying. If you have high standards for yourself and don't want to try something until you're perfect, you will put things off for a very long time.

The bottom line is to let go of trying to achieve the "best" social skills. If you wait to be perfect, you'll lose many opportunities and continue to be isolated. You won't be able to fine-tune your learning.

There is a saying (from Voltaire) "Perfection is the enemy of the good." No one is perfect or has perfect social skills. Remember that no one knows exactly how to go about these things and it's okay to make mistakes. In fact it can be a good thing, as making a few mistakes and being just good enough creates a connection with others. The important thing is to try and take the risk of being imperfect. Learn to observe and then give yourself permission to be human and perfectly imperfect!

Using Social Skills to Make Connections

As mentioned earlier, you may avoid reaching out for a variety of reasons. Now let's dig a little deeper. When you know what specific problems stand in your way of making social connections, you can learn a social skill to solve them.

PROBLEM: *Your Thoughts Get in the Way*

In Chapter 5 you learned to be aware of how negative thoughts about yourself and how others see you can get in the way of many aspects of living well. When you want to make more connections with others, it's also important to be aware of and counteract unrealistic thoughts about other people. Negative thoughts about the social situations themselves can also create obstacles.

- *I am lonely and have no friends. I'm such a loser—why would anyone want to associate with me?*
- *I hate networking events—I never know what to talk about. They are meaningless and trivial.*
- *Most people only want to talk about themselves and their accomplishments. They are not interested in me.*

These are strong statements that will lead to anxious, sad, or angry feelings and further negative thoughts about yourself. "I am lonely" expresses an emotion, whereas "I have no friends" is either a fact or an overgeneralization. Lots of different thoughts about social connections can contribute to isolation, and changing them is vital to living well.

SOLUTION: *Examine Your Thoughts*

The following suggestions will help you apply many of the skills from Chapter 5 specifically to making social connections.

• **Use a thought record.** Identify a specific situation that occurred today. Complete a thought record and identify any thoughts that make you feel bad or lead to avoidance. Are any of these thoughts unrealistic?

• **Catch any labels such as "loser."** Would you say that word out loud to anyone else? It's mean, hurtful, and does not lead to any solutions. It may lead you to want to give up and stay alone. Ditch the label and stick to the facts (clue: pejorative labels are never facts).

• **Look at any questions that you have posed.** ("Why would anyone talk to me?" "What should I talk about at a networking event?" "How can I prevent myself from being taken advantage of?") Virtually all "why?" questions are not helpful at all, as it's very difficult to answer them. ("Why am I such a loser?" "Why does no one like me?") Change them into fact-based questions, such as "How can I shift the loser label?" Questions such as "how?" or "what?" questions that lead to answers and potential solutions can be helpful. For example, "What should I talk about?" can be answered by coming up with ideas of things to talk about at an event. Unanswered questions escalate anxiety, so be sure to respond to them in your thought record.

• **Look at the evidence realistically.** While some people do not have friends, most of us have people in our lives ranging from acquaintances, to people that we know in specific situations, to closer friends.

• **Consider the people in your life.** Is there anyone you consider an acquaintance? Do you see some people regularly at places that you go to such as a coffee shop, church, or family get-togethers? Is there anyone that you're interested in getting to know better? Identify a specific person that you could talk to and take action.

PROBLEM: *You Feel Invisible*

- *No one notices me. I hate being looked at. While I have worked hard to blend into the crowd, it's discouraging and makes it difficult to connect with others.*

- *I want to have friends but worry so much that I'm not good enough that I'm terrified to say anything. When I do speak up, I'm so hesitant and quiet, no one listens anyway. I'll probably say something stupid.*

People who are socially anxious work hard not to be the center of attention, trying to blend in and responding and reacting rather than initiating. You may speak quietly or not at all. You may ensure that you wear clothing or a hairstyle that won't stand out. You caution yourself not to laugh too loudly or at the "wrong" time. You may be so successful at blending in that people truly don't notice you, or you may speak so quietly that others do not hear you. And yet others not noticing you leads to thoughts such as that what you say is not interesting or doesn't count. It hurts not to be noticed, and yet others truly may not see you if you fade into the background.

SOLUTION: *Let Yourself Be Seen*

- **Be aware of how others might see (or not see) you.** Facial expression is a crucial part of communication. Simple steps to try include looking directly at other people and scanning the room. Don't look down or avoid eye contact—it will make you look bashful, snobbish, unfriendly, or evasive. Others are less likely to approach you. If you are uncomfortable with eye contact (many people with social anxiety are), simply look around or at people's faces.

- **Try an experiment—smile!** A smile makes a difference. Don't underestimate its power! Smile regularly at people that you meet. It may feel kind of weird and unnatural, but try it anyway. Greeting someone with a smile and a slight nod is not too difficult, and you can work to make it a habit.

• **Try to be noticed.** Wear a colorful outfit or try a new hairstyle. See how many people notice—do you receive compliments or any comments? Being noticed is a good thing. It is sometimes surprising, though, what others do not notice. Have you ever received the comment "There is something different about you, but I can't put a finger on it"? The other person can't always differentiate between new eyeglasses, a new haircut, and a facial expression. Don't take it personally; some people have better observation skills than others. It's also somewhat reassuring to realize that it often takes big changes to be noticed and there's lots of room to experiment with small things.

• **Join in.** In most social situations people gravitate to those they know, making it difficult if you don't know anyone or feel anxious. It can be daunting to break into a preformed group. Standing alone in a corner is lonely. Try to physically join in; stand within earshot and close to a group. Move a bit closer. Try to appear interested in the conversation, even if it's by nodding your head and looking around at the people in the group. There may be an opportunity to make a comment, but if not, that's okay.

SOLUTION: *Let Yourself Be Heard*

• **Talk so others will listen.** You may have had others ask you to speak up or slow down. People who are socially anxious often speak very quietly and quickly. It's easy to let uncertainty creep into your tone or to include lots of pauses, *ums*, and *ahs*—all of which prevent others from understanding you or from hearing you. And then when someone else speaks up (or perhaps says the same thing you just said), it becomes easy to take offense and feel resentful. Practice speaking more loudly and slowly into a voice recorder. Imagine that you're giving a speech to an audience and articulate carefully. Be sure to look at others when you speak and speak a little bit louder and slower than you usually do.

• **Listen so others will talk.** You may pride yourself on your listening skills—many people with social anxiety do. I'm sorry to let you know that many socially anxious people are not good listeners at all. They are distracted by their own self-consciousness when they try to listen. There are blocks to listening, such as rehearsing what to say next or trying to analyze what the other person is thinking or feeling rather than truly listening. You may be thinking ahead about what to say or how to avoid questions, or you might ruminate about the many worries going through your mind. Your mind may be cluttered with thoughts about how you're coming across or predictions about what will happen next. These blocks take up space in your mind, leaving little room for listening. It's impossible to be attentive to others and worried about yourself at the same time. Learn to really listen.

• **Learn active listening.** Active listening involves not only listening to another person but also letting the person know you're listening. Look at the person and maintain eye contact and an attentive posture. Summarize and comment on or clarify what they have said, which forces you to pause and listen. An example starts with "What I heard you say was . . . . Is that right?" Ensure that you don't look away at others or at your phone during this conversation.

• **Learn the 1-2-3 steps—listening skills in action:**

1. Actively listen.
2. Respond with a summary to show that you've heard what was said.
3. Then ask a question to keep the conversation moving. Avoid questions that can be answered with one word. For example, "Do you enjoy movies?" can be answered with a yes or no, whereas "What are some of your favorite movies?" will lead to more conversation. After the other person's response, such as "I love historical drama," they are likely to ask "What about you?" which leads to the next problem—what to talk about!

PROBLEM: *You Don't Know What to Say*

• *I don't want to talk about myself—I'm not very interesting.*
• *When I talk, others will figure out that I don't know much and am pretty boring. I'd rather listen.*

Most socially anxious people are frightened to talk about themselves. Holding back feels safer as there is little opportunity for the other person to judge. You might think you're avoiding rejection and disapproval or just not being "good enough." You may be skillful at asking questions of others to avoid their asking questions of you. People who feel inadequate or uninteresting hesitate to share their thoughts and opinions and sometimes actively divert conversations to the other person. Self-disclosure can make you feel vulnerable and exposed, but it doesn't have to.

Feeling boring is not the same as *being* boring. Almost all of us have ordinary lives and ordinary interests. Relationships are built on self-disclosure, and lack of sharing often leads to being misunderstood. Remember that people are judged whether they talk or not! Learning to communicate information about yourself creates a dialogue. Self-disclosure of some type is important to keep conversations going. If you ask someone a question and they then answer it, a natural response is for you to give a similar answer. People in conversations are often searching for common ground even if it's just the weather or where they are at the time. It's okay to talk about everyday matters—most people do!

SOLUTION: *Practice Self-Disclosure*

Self-disclosure falls along a continuum. A small amount of self-disclosure can be quite straightforward and nonthreatening. It doesn't have to be intense. Examples could be your favorite color or horoscope sign. Slightly more personal information might be which part of the city you live in or your favorite television series. More personal self-disclosure can be where you were born, the number of siblings you have, or your relationship status. Of course, for some people this information could be very sensitive. For example, if your spouse recently passed away or you're alienated from your family, you might not want to talk about these issues. Very personal self-disclosure might be your opinions about reproductive rights, economic status, or hopes and goals for the future. Information about yourself that's relatively easy to share with others is a good place to start.

Self-disclosure can involve sharing facts, opinions, past experiences, and emotions. It can involve sharing how you feel in the moment, such as "When you do _____, I feel _____." The easiest type of self-disclosure involves factual, not very personal information, and the most difficult involves emotions. Take a risk—give an ordinary preference, like "I don't know about you, but I really prefer meat and potatoes to fancy fusion cuisine."

Start small and use discretion—possible areas for sharing include your interests, activities, or opinions about everyday matters. Many people are uncomfortable sharing information about their finances, sexuality, mental health, or religion, but there are big differences between people. Some people share more than others.

SOLUTION: *Think of Conversations as Trees*

Conversations start with a core or trunk and then branch out from there. It's tricky to plan what to talk about in conversations—they seem to go off in all directions. And yet they start on a main topic (the trunk of the tree) and go off in different directions (the big branches) and then off again (the twigs or small branches). There is a logic to it. For example, someone may start talking about their job and be asked a question about it. They might then turn to how much they look forward to weekends, which then turns to their leisure activities, which then turns to vacation plans. That then turns to past travel stories and goes on from there. Even if you don't like sharing stories, many people do. If you remember the image of a tree, you can consider how to branch off.

• **Consider common topics.** What do you have in common with most people you encounter? Certainly the weather, the place where you are at the moment (even if it's virtual!), local events or news items, traffic, sports, the arts, or the upcoming weekend. Think about where you are and what you share with others. It may not be particularly interesting, but it's a joining point.

• **Learn to chat.** Chitchat is simply talking about everyday matters with other people in a common setting. It's a way of finding the branch of the tree and what you share with each other. We are looking for things that we have in common when we meet others.

• **Be curious.** Ask questions. It may feel a bit intrusive, but try to find out something about the other person—they probably will appreciate it. Share something similar about yourself.

• **Learn to shift the topic.** Sometimes people talk about topics that you know nothing about or are uncomfortable with. Shifting the topic is like going off on a tree branch—it's connected but not the same. For example, if the person you are with brings up a recent hockey game that you didn't see and you have no interest in, gently shift to a similar but different topic. "I didn't see the game as I was watching . . . ." Or "I prefer watching tennis." Or "I don't know how to skate, but I like swimming."

• **Learn to move on.** Once you get started in a conversation, it can be difficult to know how to end it and leave or move on to someone else. Appropriate endings include polite comments, such as "I've enjoyed talking to you, but I need to talk to XXX." If others are there, shift your attention to someone else and ask them a question. Many people make an excuse such as "I need to use the restroom" or "I need to get a drink."

PROBLEM: *You Worry about Making Mistakes*

• *What if my mind goes blank? If I'm introducing people, what if I can't remember their names?*

• *I'm going to stutter and make mistakes.*

• *I've been told that I apologize a great deal—I have found myself saying "Sorry" when no one else is there!*

• *I tend to talk a lot and hate empty spaces in conversations.*

Negative predictions are easy to make, but they generate anxiety, which makes mistakes more likely to happen. Almost everyone has drawn a blank during introductions or substituted the wrong word in a conversation. Have you ever noticed that the harder you try to think of the word, the less likely you will be able to? The more you focus on not making a mistake, the more likely you are to notice one.

Pauses and silences are natural during conversations. It's easy to feel the need to fill them in when you're anxious. Resist this urge. It can help to remember that you're responsible for only the portion of the conversation commensurate with how much of the group you represent. If it's just you and one other person, you carry only 50% of the responsibility; if you're one of four, you are only 25% responsible.

Anxious people tend to apologize frequently, often for things that are not at all their fault or for events that were beyond their control. Apologies tend to put you in a one-down position and may make you seem guilty and responsible even if you were not.

SOLUTION: *Reduce the Pressure*

• **Be genuine.** If you draw a blank, just say so. Most people will empathize and help you out. Don't make a big deal of it. Remember that mistakes make you seem more human. If humor is comfortable for you, make a joke of it ("Oh, I can't even remember my own name right now!").

• **Use easy methods.** For example, if you're introducing yourself or a new person to a group, it's fine to ask everyone present to introduce themselves rather than put all of the pressure on yourself. Or just use first names or use the name tags people are wearing. Learn to be flexible; there are lots of ways to achieve the same goal.

• **Try timing.** An interesting experiment is to observe and time silences, particularly if they make you quite uncomfortable. They almost always feel longer than they actually are. Timing something discreetly also will help you create some distance and feel less responsible.

• **Try counting.** Consider counting your apologies (or another habit you have) for several days (try using an app such as Counter). The results can be eye-opening because many such habitual behaviors occur without your notice.

• **Substitute different words.** Replace the words "I'm sorry" with "I sincerely apologize." Having to use the additional syllables will increase your awareness and help you resist the habit. Reserve the apologies for when you really need them.

PROBLEM: *You Hate Asking for Anything*

- *If I ask for help or information, I'll look stupid.*
- *I won't make sense anyway, so I might as well keep quiet. I can figure it out myself.*

There are lots of times when we need help. While it's easy to turn to our phones for it, sometimes there's really no substitute for an in-person question. Many of us are out of practice asking for directions, opening and closing hours, or shopping information. Sometimes we may desperately need assistance, such as in an emergency. It can be dangerous not to ask.

SOLUTION: *Just Do It!*

- **Practice.** Get in the habit of putting your phone away and asking for day-to-day information—directions, the time, hours of business. Start with service people and then anyone who is nearby.

- **Get needed information.** If you or someone in your group has allergies, it can be lifesaving to ask questions about food ingredients. Clarify and ask the waiter to check with the kitchen. If you are vegetarian or vegan, ask the necessary questions rather than rely on the menu. Sometimes you need information and it's risky not to ask. I suspect people with life-threatening allergies develop very good skills in asking for information.

- **Make odd or obvious requests.** Up the difficulty level by making unusual requests, like standing in front of the pharmacy and asking where the drugstore is. Another one is asking where you could find a very unusual ingredient—say kangaroo meat when you are not in Australia, or fresh lemongrass in a small town in North America. While the answer will almost always will be "I don't know," asking will make it easier to ask when you do need an answer.

- **Ask for and accept help.** Remember that most people really like being helpful. If you need some type of help with a task like moving boxes, putting together furniture, or studying for an exam, consider asking someone who might have those skills. They could say no, but maybe they'll say yes. If you have an emergency and someone offers to help, try to accept graciously. It's so easy to respond with an "I'm fine" after you fall down and scrape your knee! The person who offers to help is being kind.

These types of requests are closely related to the next problem, which concerns figuring out your limits and learning how to set them appropriately. Many people who are socially anxious prefer to give help rather than receive it but then struggle with saying no.

PROBLEM: *You Struggle to Set Limits and Say No*

- *I was raised to be a nice person, so I should always help others. I feel guilty if I don't.*
- *I can't say no and get taken advantage of. I'm a doormat and end up resenting other people.*
- *I work way more than my colleagues and get less recognition.*
- *I'm so sorry to get in your way. I'll move.*

Many people have difficulty setting limits and saying no to other people. You may have been raised to be "nice, kind, and helpful" to everyone. While these are positive characteristics, being nice involves being considerate of yourself as well. Remember that you are part of "everyone." It's impossible to meet everyone's needs, and we all have to make choices.

People who are socially anxious often are passive and apologetic. You may put yourself down while talking and frequently apologize even for things that are not at all your fault. You may worry and feel guilty about creating conflict and just say yes to make things easier. You put others' needs before your own. You may truly think their needs are more important than yours or not have the words to express yourself.

You probably have heard the term *assertive communication,* which involves direct communication with others to let them know what you need and want while recognizing and respecting their needs and wants. It allows you to voice your concerns *and* express respect and care for yourself, the other person, and the relationship you have (see the box below). Being assertive takes time and practice, and it's easier with some people and situations than others. Just like all of the other practice activities in this book, start small and work your way up.

What Is Assertive Communication?

You may have heard the phrase *assertiveness training* or seen a class advertised in your area. Being assertive involves learning direct communication skills to let others know what you need and want while still recognizing their needs and wants. Some people worry that being assertive is the same thing as being aggressive, but it is not. It is much more than just voicing your complaints—it allows you to express respect and care for yourself and for others. Whether you want to express affection, concern, annoyance, or anger, these skills are very useful. What does it look like in action? Think of assertion as falling in the middle of a continuum between being passive and being aggressive.

Assertiveness is a way to set your limits and say no when you need to. It involves communication that is honest and straightforward, expressing your needs, listening to others, and sometimes coming to a compromise. This type of communication puts you and the other person on an equal playing field. Whereas passive people tend to put themselves in a one-down position and aggressive people tend to put themselves in a one-up position, assertive people see others as equal to themselves. Each person has something to offer, but your job is to express yourself. No one else can!

It's a good idea to explore the situations in which you have trouble saying no so you can work on that:

- What are some requests that you could say no to?
- Is it easier to say no to someone you know or someone you don't know?
- In your family, who is the most difficult person to set limits with? Do they make you feel guilty if you do? Do they push your limits?
- Think of a time where you said yes but regretted it later. What was going on at the time?

Many people find it easier to say no to those they don't know and who are not in a position of power over them. For example, it's probably harder to say no to your boss or one of your teachers than to someone you just met. You may fear consequences such as getting a negative appraisal or grade. It can also be hard to stand up to a person that you know well because you have a shared history so you may be more prone to make assumptions about how they will respond. You may say yes just to avoid rocking the boat.

> It takes time and effort to become assertive,
> but practice helps.

SOLUTION: *Start with an I Statement and Then Shift to the Other Person*

Step 1. Focus on yourself and describe to the other person what you feel, think, or need. This statement helps other people understand you and may make them feel closer to you. It can help you set limits such as "I feel put down when I'm insulted" or "I feel taken advantage of when asked to take on another task." Setting limits such as these lets others know that you have self-respect.

I statements tend to be more well received than *you* statements, which put others on the defensive. Consider the difference between "I feel upset" and "You upset me." Communicating that you feel hurt or upset clearly is scary but is often well received.

An *I* statement can simply be "I'm not interested" or "I do not need that product" when faced with a pushy salesperson. Remember there is no need to apologize, as doing so puts you in a one-down position. ("I'm so sorry that I can't take that on" may lead to a future request, especially if you say "Maybe next time"; "I don't need that service now" might be received similarly.)

Step 2. Follow up with a focus on the other person and the relationship. Say you're interested in understanding them and what their needs are. Check out any assumptions that you might be making. A simple question after your *I* statement might be "What do you think?" Another question might be "Have you checked with anyone else?" Remember that it's easier for people to make requests of those who always agree and who tend to work hard and follow through! The person making the request might be perfectly okay with asking some-one else instead. Showing them that you appreciate their confidence in you (if that is true) but are not able to help out is important. Let them know that you value the relationship.

Consider who "owns" the problem and don't take it on if you don't. It's not your responsibility to solve other people's problems, although you may choose to offer suggestions.

Here's an example: You are asked to stay late after work to help with a project you've already put a great deal of time into. You have tickets to a show that you've looked forward to and spent a lot of money on. Here is how you might respond by using first an *I* statement and then a *you* statement:

Step 1. I am not able to stay late this evening. I have spent a lot of time working these past few weeks and have plans to go to a show that I'm looking forward to.

Step 2. I know that this project is important to our work group and there are deadlines to be met. I appreciate your confidence in me, and I have learned a great deal. I know that X and Y are also in the group, I wonder if they might be available.

As noted above, it's not your job to solve the problem for your supervisor or boss, but it's helpful at times to offer suggestions or alter-natives. It demonstrates that you want to help solve the problem but also recognizes that you don't *own* the problem.

It's much easier to say no to an unreasonable request, particularly if it's impossible to accept. See these as opportunities to practice. Exam-ples might be "Can I borrow $10,000?" or "Can I take your new car on a road trip for the next two weeks?" A suitable response to these might be simply "I am not able to do that." Overexplaining is a slippery slope—"I don't have the money right now" can lead to a request for a smaller amount or "When do you think you might have it?" "I need the car this week to drive to work" may lead to "I can put my road trip off by a couple of weeks." It's more effective to minimize any justification you might want to offer for turning down these types of requests. Once again, watch the apologies!

Amira was excited about a job interview she was going to have the following week. She was spending time preparing by researching the company and rehearsing interview skills with a job coach. Her mother called her to let her know that she had a medical appointment the following week with a specialist and she really needed Amira to come with her to ask questions and record the answers. She said she was counting on her. The appointment was scheduled for the same day as the interview. Amira's brother was typically very busy with his job and family and not available.

What could Amira say to her mother? Her answers could include "I know that I've taken you to appointments many times, and I know that you've appreciated my support. I have a job interview the same day as the appointment, and I cannot change it. Your health is important to me, but I will not be able to take you. Can we think of other solutions?" With these answers Amira would be supportive but clear. Potential solutions could be Amira's mother going on her own in a taxi, asking a friend to accompany her, trying to change the appointment time, or asking her son (Amira's brother). As Amira doesn't own this problem, it's important that she offer help but not solve the problem for her mother. For example, Amira's mother should ask someone else or call to change the appointment herself.

Amira had already intended to set up a meeting with her brother, but this dilemma gave her the push to do it immediately. She called him and asked to meet on the weekend in a coffee shop. During this meeting she presented the situation with their mother as a joint family issue. He said he was very busy, but when pushed to share the issues, he had some suggestions such as asking another family member to be involved or paying for a support person. He was not opposed to occasionally driving their mother as long as he could book the appointments into his schedule well in advance. Amira left the meeting pleased that she had had the courage to assert herself rather than continue to be resentful.

Moving Forward

In this chapter you've learned about many aspects of communication and tools that you can try out for yourself. Be patient and practice one step at a time. In the midst of a conversation, you won't be able to remember all of these details. Go easy on yourself, and if you master a few new skills over time, that's great! A very important piece to remember is to try to let yourself make mistakes and be imperfect. The next two chapters offer strategies you can use in problem areas that typically arise in important areas of your life—friends, family, and partners as well as work and school.

navigating your personal life— friends and family

In Chapter 7 you learned and practiced the basics of communication skills and making connections with other people. With practice, those skills can enhance your relationships, an important part of living well. But anxiety can sometimes make it difficult to call up new tools when you need them most—in those sticky situations that we all occasionally find ourselves in with friends, family, and partners. So this chapter offers specific ways to apply those skills to common relationship problems. The more you use your skills, the more automatic they become, and the less your social anxiety is likely to interfere in your quality of life.

The problems targeted in this chapter are encountered by many socially anxious people and others, and they are by no means the only ones you may face. But the solutions have worked for many people in many circumstances, and they provide adaptable strategies that will allow you to tackle your fears with courage and curiosity. As you try out the strategies, assess how they help you and tweak them to suit your own interactions. If something doesn't work as well as you would like, modify it or try something else! What's important is to keep trying—patience and persistence will pay off.

Creating and Maintaining a Community of Friends

Human beings long to belong to some type of community, whether it's a friend or peer group, a club or faith group, a neighborhood, or a mental health peer group. People may belong to multiple communities. Our cities tend to be anonymous places, and loneliness is a widespread problem contributing to mental health problems. There has been an increase in virtual communities, as it's much easier to find people with similar interests or beliefs through online searches and groups. These communities are helpful and part of the solution to loneliness. We do, however, also need and want in-person contact to have a full life. The question is how to develop it.

> It's human to long to belong.

I Don't Know Where to Begin—I'm All Alone

Reading this book and practicing the skills and strategies taught in the preceding chapters *is* a beginning! Everyone has some people in their lives. It's a question not of where to begin but of how to increase and enrich your relationships. This is not only a less overwhelming question but a more accurate one.

PROBLEM: *I Don't Have a Group of Friends*

While you surely know some people, you may not have the friends you want or the people you can call to do things with or to support you when needed. You may have contacts with people from different parts of your life—school, work, or a group that pursues a certain common interest. But you've seen these people only in that context, they don't know each other, and you don't call on them for support. How can you connect the dots to form a community?

SOLUTIONS

- **Think about the connections you have.** Is there anyone you already know that you'd like to get to know better or see more often? Think about what you might have in common with them even if it's a small thing, like living in the same building.

- **Make connections with people you know.** A useful exercise is to make regular contact with someone you know by text, email, or just by acknowledging them when you run into each other. Make an effort to use the skills that you've learned. Practice making small talk and being friendly. If it's someone you know but have not communicated with in a while, why not reach out and see how they're doing?

- **Spend more time in public spaces.** Most libraries have computer workstations or reading areas, or provide educational activities such as presentations or classes. Most cities have festivals, sporting events, or other activities that are inexpensive or free. It's fine to go on your own as there will be lots of people around. Even saying hello to people at the grocery store or supermarket can lead to short conversations or discussions.

- **What are your interests?** Do some research on what is available in your area. Sign up for an interest group or activity. Most cities have Meetup groups (*meetup.com*), which are intended to help people connect with others who have similar interests. If you're not sure what you would like to do, try something new or unique—you never know, you just might like it! Rather than make a commitment, go to an evening activity or lecture. If it appeals to you, go again.

- **Go to one of the groups for an in-person meeting.** It will be difficult the first time or two, but regular attendance will help you feel more comfortable. Consider whether or not the people there could become friends over time.

Ryan started attending an in-person gaming group. At first he dreaded going and mostly went to keep his mother off his back. He avoided eye contact and settled into the first gaming station near the exit door. Despite his efforts to avoid others, however, they tended to cluster around and watch him play. Over a few months he became more comfortable, particularly when he realized that he was very skilled at the games and received positive feedback from others. He started learning others' names and greeted them when he arrived. As he was leaving one day, he had the realization that he had things in common with the other young people there and he looked forward to going. He saw a notice advertising an upcoming competition with cash prizes and considered signing up.

PROBLEM: *How Do I Take the Next Step?*

How do you move from being a classmate or acquaintance to becoming a friend? That step usually requires talking to and seeing others outside the place where the group meets. It can happen naturally— for example, in a work or classroom setting, people sometimes leave together, meet up for study sessions, or congregate at a coffee shop close by. But it often takes time and effort to figure out how to take the next step.

SOLUTIONS

• **Focus on possibilities.** As you've already learned, many people with social anxiety focus inwardly and may not notice when others are interested in them or when opportunities arise. Ryan decided to enter the game competition, partly as he knew he was skilled and was motivated by the potential prizes. The potential reward outweighed the social risk. Be sure to observe others and your environment to see the possibilities that might already be there.

• **Be brave.** Taking the next steps to get to know others in a different context or setting requires courage. Safe risks, such as the one that Ryan is going to try, are a good way to do it. Sometimes you may have to just put yourself out there and extend the connection into other environments, such as asking for someone's contact information, help with a problem, or walking along with them to a transit stop. Moving from one setting to another is a great step forward. Your automatic thoughts might be that you will be rejected or the other person might ignore you, but you will never know unless you try.

- **Take the initiative.** Most people with social anxiety wait for invitations rather than make them. What is the worst that could happen? A no leaves you in the same position as before you asked, and you can try asking someone else!

- **Be specific.** Many people give general invitations such as "Let's go for lunch sometime" rather than "Do you have time for coffee after class next Wednesday?" It's easy for general invitations to be interpreted as a kind of insincere gesture; often they never happen. In such cases the invitee might be left confused and wondering what happened. If it's the last time you might see someone (such as the final class or a one-time presentation), ask for their contact information to signal your genuine interest.

- **Repeat!** Forming friendships takes time, and people with social anxiety are likely to take longer than others. Sign up for activities where you will see the same group of people over an extended period. Most friendships form in places like school, college, or work, where people see each other often and over time.

- **Consider volunteerism.** Another possibility for meeting people is volunteer work. Find something you would like to do and ensure that it involves being with other people. You will provide some community service and may get free admission to events and meet like-minded people. Ideas include local arts or sporting events, a food bank, civic politics, a school, or seniors center. If you have a particular skill set, you likely will be in great demand.

- **Consider clubs.** Don't follow Groucho Marx's advice: "I refuse to join any club that would have me as a member." Most towns and cities have a variety of groups and clubs. Go to activities where you think you might meet friendly and interesting people.

- **Look for specialty groups.** Social anxiety (or other mental health) support groups can be very helpful and a good way to meet other people with similar issues. Some of them organize social outings for practice and social support. Another idea is Toastmasters International (*toastmasters.org*), which is intended to help with confidence and build public speaking skills. It is reputed to have a very supportive atmosphere, and most locations have a choice of groups. I have had many clients attend Toastmasters after treatment for social anxiety, with the aim of continuing to practice skills as well as to meet others.

> **PRACTICE EXERCISE: The list**
>
> Make a list of 10 different people you know from different walks of life. They may be people that you have not talked to in a long time. Do some research to figure out their contact information—this step is remarkably easy with Google, Facebook, and other social media platforms. Contact them one by one just to say hello and ask them how they are. Don't take it personally if you don't get an answer since it's impossible to be sure they received the message or that you got the correct person. If they respond, try to engage in some chitchat to catch up. You never know, an old friendship might be reactivated or a new one begun. Keep working your way down the list. If you hit the end, start a new list!

Is It Worth the Effort?

Once friendships are formed, they can bring their own set of complications. At times it can be tempting to just walk away and avoid conflict or difficulties. It's important, however, to learn not only how to begin and form relationships but also to address problems within the relationships when they occur.

PROBLEM: *What Can I Do about a Friend Who Is Taking Advantage?*

Healthy relationships generally feel reciprocal rather than one-sided. However, people who have low self-esteem tend to put themselves down and may do things to be liked and accepted by others, which may throw the relationship out of balance. For example, imagine that you have had a friend for a long time and, as you are working on building your confidence, you start to realize that you give more than you receive in the friendship. Because you have a car and she doesn't, you're the one who drives. A long time ago, she offered to pay for gas, but you declined, and she hasn't offered again. She expects you to pick her up and recently complained that you were a few minutes late. You tend to defer to her opinions about restaurants to go to or what activities to do, so she has gotten into the habit of making the decisions without your input. You're starting to feel resentful even though you can see that you've played a part in creating this problem. You are starting to wonder if she really likes you or just wants your help or to have someone to boss around.

SOLUTIONS

- **Be self-aware.** Many people with social anxiety have similar difficulties due to low self-esteem. These problems develop gradually, sometimes without either person in the relationship really paying attention. It becomes a habit and "just how we do things," and then becomes difficult to change. Early awareness reduces the likelihood of these types of bad habits developing.

- **Speak up.** I know this is easier said than done! Start gradually such as by stating your preference for a restaurant, an activity, or a change in the ways you interact. These requests may be easier than asking for payment for gas. If your car is in the shop, you could suggest that both of you take public transit. Or you could point out the increase in the price of gas and directly ask for a contribution.

- **Be direct.** Some people who attempt to be assertive end up being vague and subtle, hoping that the other person will pick up what they mean, but run the risk that the other person completely misses the point. Contrast the statement "I'm aware that gasoline prices have gone up. I know that I turned your kind offer down a while back but I have reconsidered and would appreciate it if you'd contribute to the cost" versus "Haven't gas prices gone up a lot? My salary hasn't kept pace with inflation."

- **Reconsider.** There are times when you start to make changes and become aware that you are being taken advantage of, so you step back and reconsider your relationships. Most of the time when you make a direct request and stand up for yourself, the other person will follow through. The relationship will feel more reciprocal. There are times, however, when this does not happen, and after several requests you might decide to pull back from the friendship. Even though it's difficult, it helps to let the other person know. If you can, tell them how their behavior has affected you and why you're pulling back. They may reconsider.

Navigating the World of Romance

Dating and befriending someone are very similar. In fact many have said that it's very important to form a friendship first with a potential romantic partner. That allows you to get to know them slowly and takes some of the pressure off. Similar skills are involved, many of which you have already learned and practiced. The risks, however, can feel greater with dating. You may feel more vulnerable forming an intimate relationship with someone and have a greater fear of rejection. But it's sad to go through life without taking the risks involved!

Dating

Many people use online dating apps to meet others, which certainly can make it easier and reduce some of the early steps of finding someone you might be compatible with. But I've noticed that these profiles often overemphasize interests: "I love to travel and walk on the beach while watching the sunset." While interests are important, so are common values, beliefs, and more subtle factors such as a similar sense of humor. The importance of the ability to communicate and laugh at each other's jokes and foibles can't be overestimated. People who "get" each other will enjoy their time spent together. Feeling understood by another human being is a crucial part of relationships.

PROBLEM: I Want to Ask Someone on a Date

Maybe you've chatted with someone who works in your office a few times while coming into the building. You don't know them well, but they seem friendly. You find yourself thinking about them and realize you're attracted to them. You'd like to get to know them better.

SOLUTION: *Just Do It!*

Start small but get specific. There are lots of possibilities and questions. Do you know their name? It can be awkward to ask after numerous conversations, but go for it. Say something like "I feel that I should know this already, but I realize I don't know your name" after you introduce yourself. You can then ask for their contact information, even if it may be readily available if the two of you work for the same employer. A small step could be "I'd like to continue our conversation—how about if we meet up in the lunchroom at noon today?" Another next step could be proposing lunch at a restaurant nearby, progressing to a drink after work on a Friday. With each step, the two of you are getting to know each other better and seeing what you have in common.

PROBLEM: *I Want to Get Closer to Someone I've Been on a Date With*

Once you've gone on a date with someone, your interest in them may be piqued and you decide that you'd like to get to know them better. You want to see them again and even become close to them. It can be tricky to figure out what to do next and waiting does not always work out!

SOLUTION: *Take a Risk*

This part of a new relationship can feel quite risky, as it involves figuring out a way to let the other person know that you are interested. In general, it's best to take small steps and start to consider what you have in common. These may be interests, similar backgrounds, or activities. You could take the bull by the horns and suggest a second date. Or at minimum, send a text after the first date and let the person know that you enjoyed meeting them and hope that you can get together again.

Jody had been on three dates with Bill after meeting him through an online dating app. Her friend Emily advised her to take it slow, first meeting in a public place for coffee, next going for a walk that ended with ice cream, and then having dinner at a local Italian restaurant. Jody was shy, but when Bill shared that he tended to be shy as well, she felt much more comfortable. She realized that they might have things in common. It felt awkward initially, but they managed to find things to talk and laugh about. They both grew up in a smallish city and had two siblings. They shared some of the same experiences when they moved to the larger city for work. They realized they enjoyed the same type of movies and music. Bill tentatively suggested they go to an upcoming music festival that would require an overnight stay in a nearby city.

Bill clearly wanted to become closer to Jody. Myriad thoughts went through her mind when he made this overture, and she didn't know what to say. She stumbled on her words and said she'd have to think about it. His request brought up many questions: whether they'd be able to continue to find things to talk about over the course of two days, how the sleeping arrangements would work, whether he was implying they might become intimate, and who would pay for the tickets, the food, and the hotel. There was so much to navigate that Jody was tempted to decline. Over the next few days she carefully thought about his invitation and decided she wasn't ready. She was, however, interested in getting to know Bill better and worried that he might feel rejected if she said no. She looked for other alternatives and found out there was a concert in town in a few weeks featuring a musician they both liked. She called Bill that evening and proposed the alternative, and he eagerly accepted.

Jody was pleased with how she'd handled the situation. Rather than saying no and retreating as usual because she felt overwhelmed and anxious, she was able to develop her relationship with Bill while choosing an option that made her feel more in control.

PROBLEM: Should I Tell the Person I'm Dating That I Experience Social Anxiety?

"Should I, when do I, or how do I disclose personal information such as mental health status or any other problems such as medical conditions?"

is a question I've been asked often. The answer is that it depends on the situation and the individuals involved. Obviously, if you meet someone in a social anxiety support group, the discussion is moot. Disclosing personal information requires trust; see the box below.

The Components of Trust

It can be difficult to place your trust in another human being. To trust someone can lead to feelings of vulnerability. You may have had your trust betrayed in the past if someone made fun of you or shared your personal story with someone else. Most people who are socially anxious struggle to trust others as they fear judgment. And yet trust is crucial for the development of relationships. Trust must be built over time with another person, so be patient. It also requires you to share parts of yourself with others and take a risk. It's scary!

It helps to think of trust as multifaceted. You don't have to—and shouldn't, in most cases—place complete trust in a single person regarding all matters. Answer the following questions:

- Who would you trust to fix your car?
- Who would you ask to help you move between apartments?
- Who would you trust for medical advice?
- Who would you call if you had an emergency such as a fire in the middle of the night (after calling 911)?
- If you urgently needed $500, who could you ask?
- If you won the lottery, who would you call first?
- Who would you call on for emotional support?
- Who have you shared your difficulties with social anxiety with?
- Who have you asked for personal advice, and provided personal advice to?

You can see from these questions and your answers that you trust some people for some things but not for others—a therapist for emotional support but hopefully not to fix your car, someone to help you move furniture but not to be a confidant, and so on. You may also trust a certain person for one quality but not another, such as a coworker to be reliable but not necessarily competent. Trust is multifaceted.

SOLUTIONS

- **Don't be too quick to disclose**—certainly not on the first date. You may want to just get it over with as you worry about rejection, but you want to ensure that the other person knows you a bit so has a chance to respond to you as a person and not just to your mental health status.

- **Seize the moment.** If the two of you are talking about personal matters and the other person discloses something, you can listen with empathy and then consider whether it's a good time to reciprocate. Sharing personal information builds closeness.

- **Be realistic and accurate.** You could share your diagnosis if you've had one, or say you've wondered whether you should see a professional or that you've read some books like this one and relate to them. If you've had treatment, you might mention some improvements you've experienced, such as being on a date. Don't catastrophize ("I'm never going to get better") or minimize ("It's no big deal").

- **Paint yourself as a whole person.** Besides the problems and successes you've had with social anxiety, be sure to share other parts of yourself. You're not just someone with a diagnosis.

- **Ask for discretion.** Let the other person know that you're divulging this personal information because you trust them and value the relationship. Be very clear what you want and expect regarding your disclosure. While discretion cannot be guaranteed, it's wise to ask them not to share this information with anyone else.

- **Prepare to be surprised.** You may, like many of my clients, be anxious and fear judgment and possible rejection when you share your mental health experiences. Yet almost everyone can relate to social anxiety and its symptoms. Mental health has been discussed extensively in the media, and most people either have their own stories to share or know someone with similar issues. Being open about these issues opens the door to more closeness and sharing, with friends, partners, and family.

Endings and Beginnings

It's impossible to predict the direction any relationship will take. Some end. Some present a new beginning. Anxiety may come up no matter how a relationship evolves.

PROBLEM: *My Relationship Has Ended*

The situation you've feared has happened—a person you've been dating has said they've decided to move on. Even if you've been picking up some clues of waning interest, you may feel shocked and embarrassed that you didn't see it coming. It's difficult not to take it personally even if you were offered the classic "It's not you, it's me" reassurance and no other reasons for the breakup.

SOLUTIONS

- **Allow yourself to be sad.** It's perfectly normal to be sad when relationships end, particularly if it wasn't your choice and you would have preferred to keep dating this person. One of the great ironies in life is that you have to be willing to be rejected to find true intimacy.

- **Reach out for support.** This is a good time to share with a trusted friend. If you haven't had much experience in this area, you might not realize that almost everyone has had relationships end and shares your experience.

- **Complete a thought record (or two).** It's important to keep your automatic thoughts in check and to dampen down tendencies to blame yourself. It's normal to rehash your last few times together to try to figure out what happened. And unless the other person told you, it's impossible to know for sure.

- **Put it in perspective.** How serious was the relationship? While any breakup will be difficult and maybe even heartbreaking, a relationship that you've been in for a few weeks or months is different than one of several years.

- **Treat yourself well.** You may want to punish and berate yourself with your thoughts, but be kind. You did, after all, take the risk of being in a relationship and probably learned lots of things along the way. Taking risks means you are brave.

- **Resist an urge to avoid.** Some clients call this urge "turtling," or withdrawing into your shell. If you experience this urge, set a time limit and push yourself out of it after a day or two.

PROBLEM: *I'm Getting Married!*

The other end of the spectrum! In fact, many of us would not think of this as a problem. This happy news is very exciting but can lead to lots of different kinds of stressors for people with social anxiety. If your fiancé wants a big traditional wedding, you may dread being the center of attention, eating in front of people at the head table, and having all eyes on you during a "first dance." I have had clients come to see me specifically for help in navigating their wedding—one in particular had an intense fear of saying his vows at the altar with his back facing the guests. His automatic thought was that others would be snickering and making fun of him. Then there are the matters of speeches, money, gifts, and who to (and not to!) invite. Family and friend pressures often come into play and can sometimes create conflict for the couple. The temptation might be to elope.

SOLUTIONS

- **Communicate with your partner.** Be clear about what vision each of you has for the wedding day. Your visions may be quite different, and both of you will likely have to compromise. It's important to do this early so you're on the same page before families get involved in the planning. Talk often and openly. While it may sound unromantic and businesslike, it can help to keep notes or create a spreadsheet for the wedding planning.

- **Communicate with your families.** Often social challenges at weddings are instigated by family members. They may have opinions about who "has to" be invited or where the wedding should take place. If the family is paying for some or all of the wedding day, you may think they have the right to dictate events. Your parents may want to invite their friends and distant relatives, which affect financial and other considerations such as location. Again, open and frequent dialogue is important. Clarify your bottom line on issues that really matter to you, but be flexible where you can. Families all have their own traditions and cultural expectations for weddings and other life events.

• **Review the principles of assertive communication (see Chapter 7).** When making plans including other people and all are excited and want to be involved, it will be crucial to set limits so that things don't get out of hand. Emotions can run high. You and your fiancé may have to be firm. Have everyone agree to resolutions of disagreements in public so that all are clear and misunderstandings don't happen.

• **Keep it simple.** Weddings can cost a great deal of money and create stress for everyone, and there's something to be said for simplicity. Some of the most memorable weddings may be held in a backyard or at a local park with a food truck. Ditching a formal wedding can also reduce your social anxiety as you are likely to feel less anxious in a casual setting. Now is not the time to be a hero and conquer your social anxiety!

• **It's okay to use safety behaviors.** If there is a time to help reduce your anxiety in some subtle ways (see Chapter 6), it might be on your wedding day. For example, the client who didn't want his back to the congregation during his vows asked to stand facing his fiancé so that he could not only look at her but glance at others as well. He felt less vulnerable and anxious. If there is going to be a first dance, ensure that others are asked to join in quickly so that you and your partner are alone on the dance floor for only a brief time.

• **Preparation.** If a banquet, speeches, and dancing are going to be an important part of the day, plan ahead and prepare. Practice your vows and speech until you feel confident. Up the ante—start on your own, record yourself, and then have a small audience. Take dance lessons—many couples do.

- **Embrace imperfection.** No event is perfect, and there is joy to be found in mistakes and imperfection. These events are what create memories and stories over the years. For example, "choking up" and needing a moment to finish your vows will actually endear you to others.

- **Avoid alcohol.** While this advice may sound like a fun-killer, it will help you stay on top of the situation. Alcohol acts as a depressant drug, so if you drink too much you will become disinhibited and may say and do things that you regret later. While it's fine to do the toasts, keep it to a minimum at least until the speeches and formal parts of the event are over.

Navigating Family Life

Navigating family life with social anxiety brings up many considerations thanks to the mind-boggling number of variables involved. You may have family members who also struggle with social anxiety, and that seems "normal" for all of you. Or others may be outgoing and comfortable in social situations, so you feel like the odd person out. You have known your family all your life, so you have a vast collection of shared experiences. Each family member may have a certain "role," and you may expect them to always behave the same way they have in the past. It can be hard to break out of longtime patterns with family members. Longstanding "jokes," barbs, teasing, and much more can lead you to dread gatherings for fear of being hurt or embarrassed once again. With the following scenarios and suggestions how to cope with them, I've tried to capture some common dilemmas but can't be comprehensive. Hopefully, these ideas will get you started on navigating family interactions with less anxiety.

PROBLEM: *Help—I'm Going Home for Thanksgiving!*

All families have positive and negative holiday patterns. Just as for big events such as weddings, when families are together for holidays emotions can be intense. You may find yourself reverting to old patterns and ways of relating to parents when you return to the family home, especially if you are sleeping in your childhood bedroom! They may continue to see you as a child rather than the adult you have become. Issues of responsibilities for food and hosting, money, alcohol, or political discussions can easily come up. Tensions often come to the forefront, and people may not enjoy the holiday as much as they would like. Here are some solutions that may increase your comfort and reduce your anxiety.

SOLUTIONS

- **Set the expectations before arriving.** Let your family members know what you plan to bring and about any changes in your life. For example, Jody went back to her home city for Christmas and decided to bring Bill along. She let her parents know in advance that he would be coming and that they would be sharing a bedroom. She didn't ask for permission and worked hard to sound confident when she shared the information.

- **Suggest a new tradition.** If there has tended to be a lot of alcohol consumption at family gatherings or everyone falls asleep after dinner in front of the television, announce to whoever might be interested that you would like to go for a walk, play an outdoor game, or set up a board game competition in the basement. It's helpful to plan this alternative activity in advance, perhaps by making arrangements with a cousin or sibling. You never know whether your family has been waiting for an injection of new energy into the holiday traditions!

- **Increase structure and participation.** While it can be difficult to do this when you're not the host, structure and activities help with the quiet times and will be more fun. Talk to your parents about this idea in advance and they might appreciate it. It's easy for the hosts to work very hard with food and other preparations in advance and during the day itself and end up exhausted and resentful. Having everyone participate in some way, by contributing a dish, helping with cleanup, or just taking the dog for a walk, may just work.

• **Keep it light.** If you notice that others are talking about difficult topics (see the next section) or about family issues from the past, gently change the topic or work to lighten the mood.

• **Retain perspective.** While you may try these suggestions and some of them may help, it can be difficult to shift long-established traditions. If the situation ends up being very draining and tiring, consider taking strategic breaks by going to your bedroom, calling a friend, or even leaving early. There are also times when family events can be not just negative but even toxic and damaging to your growth. If there is a history of past abuse or high levels of conflict in your family, consider whether to attend in the future. You have no obligation to harm yourself to preserve traditions.

PROBLEM: *I Don't Know How to Talk about Controversial Topics*

Most of us agree that the world has become more divisive than it used to be and it's difficult to have conversations about controversial topics. It's easy to create conflict without intending to, and people may be sensitive to certain words or types of language. People with social anxiety often struggle to state their opinion for fear of being negatively evaluated, and changes in our society can add a layer of complication.

SOLUTIONS

• **Start with neutral topics.** If you're talking with someone whose opinions you're not familiar with or whom you haven't seen in a while, start with (hopefully) neutral topics such as local events, family vacations, or memorable activities.

• **Test the water.** When you're not sure, ask rather than wade into uncharted territory. Ask questions such as "Is it okay to talk about world events?" or "Are you planning to vote in the upcoming elections?" Hopefully, the answer will be positive, which can lead to an interesting discussion.

• **Agree to disagree.** When it's clear that there are family divides over certain issues, try to have everyone agree that it's not going to be a useful discussion and will not lead to a positive outcome. Just say something like "I respect your opinion. I don't agree with you, however, and prefer not to discuss it further." Or, "Let's agree to disagree."

- **Change the topic.** This can be done in either a straightforward way ("Let's talk about something different") or in a subtle way ("That reminds me of the time . . .").

- **Leave the room.** If all else fails and it's not going well, excuse yourself and go into another room or for a walk. Becoming upset and having the occasion ruined is not worth it. Some people cannot be dissuaded from their ideas and might even goad those with different opinions. People whose opinions are widely divergent are unlikely to find common ground unless they are willing to at least try to understand another point of view.

PROBLEM: *A Family Member Has Asked for Financial Help*

Jorge had numerous cousins, all of whom lived in the same city. Luis was two years younger than Jorge and frequently had business schemes. He was trained as a chef but wasn't very good with money. He'd lost money investing in a restaurant but remained very optimistic. Jorge was slowly saving his money for a house and was deliberate and cautious with his investments. Just after a relaxed lunch that Jorge had paid for, Luis brought out some documents that laid out a business plan for buying a food truck. He asked Jorge to invest $15,000 and was confident that he'd either pay it back in a year or Jorge could be a partial owner. Luis said that he was planning to approach other family members, but he wanted Jorge to have the "first opportunity."

Money is a tricky topic, particularly in the context of family loyalties. It's often easier to say no to someone who you don't know well, or to make an excuse as they may not know much about your income or resources. Saying no to a family member often leads to guilt, particularly if you believe you should always help out your family. You may be worried that you'll insult the other person, hurt their feelings, or get an indignant and angry response to your saying no. You may, however, know their history better than most and have a strong premonition that you'll not only fail to make a profit but end up getting no money back at all. Jorge wants to say no.

SOLUTIONS

- **Be transparent.** Jorge could let Luis know that while he has a good job, he is saving money to buy a house and that goal is very important to him. If it's true, he could say that he can't afford to both save for the house and loan Luis the money and he doesn't expect that he will be able to do so any time in the near future.

- **Be honest.** He can tell Luis that while he admires his enthusiasm and dreams, he is not comfortable taking a financial risk. He can do this without undermining Luis's business acumen.

- **Offer suggestions.** I wouldn't suggest "throwing anyone else under the bus" so to speak, such as suggesting that Luis approach another family member. The suggestion of a business loan from a bank could help Jorge feel better, even though it's likely that Luis has thought of it already.

- **Say no clearly and definitely.** It would be easy for Jorge to respond with "Not right now; it's a bad time," but this would give the impression that later on might work and he's open to being asked again. It is better not to imply that you might change your mind if you actually won't.

PROBLEM: *My Mother Is Really Struggling to Live on Her Own*

Life changes, and there are transitions that will require your involvement in family situations. An aging parent with chronic health issues is just one of them. You and your siblings may not agree on what to do, or they may expect you to resolve the issues as you have tended to step up in the past. Communication about difficult issues can create tensions especially if people disagree or, in this case, if your mother does not wish to accept support. These issues arise for everyone; however, those with social anxiety tend to be more likely to take on extra burdens or struggle to set limits with others.

Amira was working full-time and doing well in her job. It had taken her a while to become comfortable with her colleagues, but she was gaining confidence. Her brother was busier than ever, traveling overseas every month, and despite good intentions was not available very often for family needs. Amira noticed her mother's increasing frailty and occasional confusion. She scheduled an assessment for her with their family physician and arranged a time when she could attend. She was shocked at the doctor's suggestion that her mother might have dementia and should be sent for further testing. She immediately called her brother, but afterward noticed her mother's tears and crumpled face. She felt terrible for not talking to her mother first about the potential diagnosis.

SOLUTIONS

- **Talk to the person directly involved.** It's very easy to talk *about* a person or a situation rather than speaking directly *to* the person. It's more anxiety provoking to be direct, and we often fool ourselves into thinking that we're talking to other, more peripherally related people first in order to figure out what to do. While it's helpful to discuss things with others in advance at times, the best person for Amira to talk to about this problem is her mother. Many people find it difficult to bring up these types of situations and talk around them or try to resolve them indirectly. For example, if Amira hired an in-home caregiver as a "gift," her mother might be confused and surprised rather than relieved.

- **Be wary of triangulation.** It's very easy to triangulate— person A talks to person B about person C. We all do this at times, but it's poor communication. Think of a time that you complained about your boss to a colleague or talked to one friend about another. While this can include straightforward information sharing or nasty gossip, it complicates matters and is not respectful to the person being discussed.

- **Get the facts.** Anxious people tend to engage in catastrophic thinking, so get the facts before acting. Sometimes our minds can make lots of predictions and then come up with solutions for all of them without knowing the information. The facts here are that Amira's mother is having difficulties, her doctor suspects dementia, and she will be assessed further. The diagnosis is not yet known.

- **Engage in problem solving.** Once the facts (or at least more certainty) are in, it's useful to consider what the problem is (define it) and then think of a range of potential solutions. It's best to do this in a group so that some creative options can be thought of. For example, Amira, her brother, and mother could do this together. After a number of solutions are brought forward, they can each be assessed further for practicality, acceptability, and so on.

- **Take a step.** It's easy under difficult circumstances to have "decision paralysis" and just ignore the problem, hoping it will go away. This is a type of avoidance, and while it temporarily reduces anxiety, it doesn't help solve the problem. A step in Amira's case could be investigating seniors' accommodations in the community, ensuring that Amira's mother is involved in the process.

Moving Forward

The joys and benefits of relationships are immeasurable, and it's useful to be able to resolve the issues that come with the territory to reduce any interference by social anxiety. The same is true for the issues that arise in your work and educational life, the topics of the next chapter.

9

navigating your professional life— school and work

Just as friend and family relationships, discussed in Chapter 8, are key to living well, so is being engaged in the world through learning and working. Unfortunately, people who are socially anxious often do not achieve their professional potential due to avoidance of the interpersonal situations involved in education and employment. When you have trouble speaking in front of others and advocating for yourself, or working with a team or collaborating in a study group, you may yield to the temptation to avoid jobs that you'd be good at and that would advance your career or to enroll only in classes that require no presentations. (I've had students decline to register for one of my classes after getting an affirmative answer to their query about whether I required presentations for the course!)

As you now know, fear of being judged is common among those with social anxiety. Being evaluated and judged is an inescapable part of having a job and getting an education. In these domains, you're not subject to merely thinking you'll be evaluated and judged; often you really are being judged—to assess whether you deserve the job you want, a raise, or a promotion, or to earn a degree or certification. The stakes can be high as your future may hinge on another person's decision. This chapter will help you develop skills to feel more confident and face these challenges head on.

On the upside, most occupational and educational environments are subject to laws, regulations, and guidelines that can remove some of the ambiguity about what kind of anxiety-provoking situations you may encounter and how you and others are expected to behave. That can be a comfort, especially when starting a new job or enrolling in a new school.

This chapter offers solutions for common problems in these two domains. As in Chapter 8, what you'll find here is just a sampling of concerns, but they should get you started. With all the social skills practice you've had in previous chapters, and the fact that you probably now know more about communication than most people, you'll be able to apply the solutions presented in the following pages to more and more situations.

> Don't let social anxiety make decisions about your future.

Charting a Course for Your Future

Employment and education give us a sense of purpose, productivity, and meaning. They help with structuring our time and provide us with a greater community with social connections. You may work or go to school to make a good living, but both employment and education can contribute more than a paycheck to your life. Which direction do you want to take—work or school?

Making a Decision

PROBLEM: *I Have No Idea What I Want to Do with My Life*

Jesse had been doing quite well at the fast-food restaurant since meeting with their boss. A positive performance appraisal and raise had not only made decent groceries and some new clothes affordable but increased Jesse's confidence to the point where they considered applying for the position of assistant manager. However, Jesse had never been in a position like that before and was terrified of the responsibility and not being able to follow through. What if they drank too much one night and slept through their alarm in the morning? What if there was a customer complaint? What if an employee got upset and left early? So many catastrophic thoughts just made them think it was a bad idea to apply. However, Jesse decided to go ahead and apply anyway.

Jesse's doubts were completely understandable, and catastrophic thoughts often lead to a decision not to do something.

Neither Jesse nor Ryan (the gamer discussed in previous chapters) had made conscious, deliberate decisions about the future. Jesse had taken the fast-food job to make enough money to move out of their parents' house. Ryan had completed high school during the pandemic and then retreated to his parent's basement and spent his nights playing online video games. Because of their tendency to be socially anxious and isolated, neither had many friends who had gone on to college. They had kept their dreams very modest, and deep down they didn't really think they'd amount to much.

It's easy to either avoid decision making or just take the steps that are immediately in front of you without deliberate planning. Actively considering your future possibilities is an act of hope and a step toward confidence in yourself.

> Start to fantasize.

SOLUTIONS

- **Consider your options:**

    1. Imagine that your social anxiety magically disappeared. What would you do? Did you fantasize about a particular career as a child? Why were you interested in it?

    2. Next, consider how social anxiety has limited your choices. Consider the major factors in the courses or jobs you've taken. Were

your choices made due to interest, availability, or lack of social challenges? Social anxiety may have been the boss and made decisions for you, rather than the other way around. If you've limited your options due to anxiety, it has been in charge!

3. Make a list. Write down at least 10 different jobs that appeal to you, or 10 different topics or courses that appeal to you. It can be hard to think of these things if you've tended to make choices on the basis of what is easy or non-anxiety-provoking. Use your imagination.

4. Narrow it down. Once you have some ideas, eliminate a few that are completely impractical (say, astronaut). What is left on the list? Any good possibilities to explore for your future?

• **Try something new.** Throughout this book, I've encouraged you to try new things, usually starting small or doing some research on a different activity. This strategy can be applied to school and work. Many of us are creatures of habit, and even driving or walking a new route that you've never taken before can help break old habits. Read about or research a topic that you've never thought about before.

• **Do information interviews.** During my career as a psychologist, I've been approached many times by high school or university students wanting to know more about my job. I've typically said yes, as it's fun to describe what I do to an interested person. Often these students didn't know a lot other than what they had seen in media portrayals.

PRACTICE EXERCISE: Information interviews

It's terrific practice to conduct an interview and be in the driver's seat. Think of a job (or an educational program) that you are interested in pursuing or learning more about. Ask others, starting with your family, if they can think of anyone you could talk to. Send the person a message and ask if you could talk to them about their job; if they are amenable, set up a time to do the interview. Create a list of questions that you would like the person to respond to. Potential questions include the educational requirements, the day-to-day activities involved, different types of opportunities, and potential for future growth. You may be in for some surprises, and even if you have minimal interest in pursuing this career, it's worth the time and effort to practice interviewing. Set up a few of these interviews, preferably in person. Be sure to send a thank you note.

The purpose of this exercise is to think about your interests, learn more about how to pursue them, and take initiative. Doing an interview with a list of questions is easier than just asking unplanned questions. Hearing about the options for different types of jobs can open up possibilities. Of course, doing interviews is also good practice for being interviewed, as you build confidence.

Navigating School

Many aspects of school can be difficult for individuals with social anxiety, particularly those involving evaluation and working with other people. Throughout this book we have touched on a number of ways to give presentations—with families, friends at school, or in work settings. Speaking up in front of others is a part of life and includes asking questions, telling jokes, making comments, as well as giving presentations. Being observed doing an activity is almost inevitable as well, depending on what the course or job is. You could be observed learning a physical skill or procedure, such as learning to do a blood draw in a laboratory technician course.

Lisa was growing bored with her job as a security guard at the mall and had been enjoying her cycling and other physical activities outside of work. She had begun exploring other options for her future after speaking to a personal trainer at a gym that she went to regularly. She discovered that there was a two-year personal trainer certificate program available at a local college and that there were the daytime classes she could attend given her evening and night shifts at the mall. She applied, even though the course required a great deal of participation and some presentations. The program also included a practicum where she would be carefully observed and rated by a qualified supervisor. Even the thought of being observed doing activities made Lisa anxious, but she enrolled after being accepted anyway.

PROBLEM: *You Will Be Observed and Graded*
by an Instructor—and Participation is Required!

As Lisa discovered, evaluation occurs in many classes or programs. Evaluation can be as informal as having the instructor track attendance, but it also can include written exams, presentations, and even oral examinations, all of which can create anxiety for shy people. The temptation might be just to forgo the marks and focus on trying to get higher grades in another assignment. This is a good example of making a decision on the basis of social anxiety. Don't do it—participation is great practice for lots of different situations.

SOLUTIONS

- **Fully show up.** Many people who are socially anxious sit near the back of class and work hard to blend in. Instead, sit closer to the front and be visible. Appear engaged and involved through your body language. If you are more noticeable, it will be easier to speak up. Nod in agreement, smile when appropriate, and look at other people.

- **Ask a question after class.** It's often easier to talk to another person one-on-one than in front of a group. Start with something factual, such as asking the instructor about an upcoming exam or readings. Ask the person sitting beside you a question about a topic being discussed.

- **Agree with someone else.** If a fellow student makes a point, say that you agree with them. It's easier to simply agree than to make a separate statement, which you can do next (for example, "I agree with you; however, I'd like to add . . .").

- **Share a brief opinion.** It's a bit easier to share an opinion by raising your hand than by responding to a question, as you are more fully in control.

- **Respond to a question.** If you have the opportunity, respond to a general inquiry, such as "Can anyone share . . . with the class?" You're less likely to be singled out if you've done this. If you are put on the spot, it's appropriate to say "I'm not sure" or "I'll have to think about it."

- **Request gradual exposure.** Some people are very uncomfortable being observed doing activities such as Lisa would have to do in a class to become a physical trainer. One possibility might be for her to let the instructor know about her circumstance so that she is not put on the spot immediately but has a chance to practice gradually with smaller tasks and then work her way up to tougher situations.

• **Repeat, repeat.** As you practice speaking up, you will gradually become more comfortable. It's great exposure for social anxiety, and it will also provide you with the participation grades for the class. This advice applies to doing any activity in front of other people: It will become easier with practice.

• **Embrace mistakes.** No one is perfect, and mistakes happen. While it can feel awkward in front of other people, saying the wrong word, giving an incorrect answer, or engaging in an incorrect move while being observed is a learning experience, and most often others are much more accepting than you are.

PROBLEM: *I've Been Assigned to Work on a Project with a Small Group*

Many people who are socially anxious prefer to work on their own rather than within a group of classmates. There are complexities to working with other people, and it's likely that the instructor has been deliberate in choosing these assignments. Many work sites require people to work within teams, so working in groups builds skills. And yet you may worry that you'll be the one who does all the heavy lifting and others will take advantage of you. That's a negative prediction and one that you will be able to influence.

SOLUTIONS

• **Keep your thoughts in check.** You likely don't know the other students well and are possibly being unfair if you are prejudging them (or yourself). Keep an open mind.

• **Use your listening skills.** When the group first meets to discuss the project, listen carefully as well as observe to get a sense of the people in the group.

• **Be forthright.** Be clear regarding your skill set (what it includes and doesn't). Remember to use the assertive communication skills you learned in Chapter 7. If there is a task that you want or don't want to take on, speak up and advocate for yourself.

• **Suggest a project plan and schedule.** Some groups are more organized than others, but it's always a good idea to have clarity and a schedule for the work involved. Be clear about your preferences and limits, even while you listen to those of others.

• **Tolerate imperfection.** Part of the difficulty in working in a group is that different people have different work styles and timelines. Only some may be prompt with their work. It can be tempting to pick up the slack, but resist the temptation! It's not your job to rescue others.

PROBLEM: *My Mind Will Go Blank*

Many people with social anxiety fear this outcome. When a person is highly anxious or even having a panic attack, it's difficult to think clearly. One variant of this is test anxiety—sitting in front of a blank screen or piece of paper without being able to think of anything remotely related to the exam. Another example might be standing in front of a classroom for your presentation and having all of your thoughts and responses seemingly fly out of your mind!

SOLUTIONS

• **Notice your thoughts.** Minds are not blank but are full of thoughts. These thoughts, however, are not necessarily the thoughts you want to have. They may be anticipatory catastrophic thoughts about the likelihood of your mind going blank, which is going to create more anxiety. Use a thought record (Chapter 5) to figure out how you might cope with whatever happens.

• **Think back to the past.** How many times has your mind gone blank before? What did you do? How did it turn out? While the outcomes may or may not have been okay, the situation was probably difficult, and it's natural to avoid thinking about stressful or embarrassing events. But it's unlikely that "all" of your thoughts really disappeared or that it happened 100% of the times that you think you are remembering. Try to determine how often these events actually happened and what exactly occurred.

- **Take a moment.** If your mind goes blank, take a few deep, slow breaths to calm down. Ground yourself in the present moment using a strategy such as clenching your fists several times. Most of the time you will feel better quickly and thoughts will start to come to mind. Remember that you can take a moment either in front of a class or at the beginning of an exam. Just pause.

- **Engage in problem solving.** What could you do? There are lots of potential strategies—if you fear your mind will go blank during a presentation, have notes or slides that can help jog your memory. Different types of study strategies can do much the same thing; consider using visualization or some type of memory trick to think of the necessary content. In oral examinations, a common strategy is to begin by repeating part of the question, as it can prime your own ideas and responses. Another idea is to preplan answers to likely questions, so that these are more readily in mind if needed.

- **Be transparent.** If you lost your train of thought or can't recall a word or phrase, say so. Most people can relate to momentary blocked thoughts. If appropriate, make a joke about it, such as "I sometimes even forget who I am!"

- **Request accommodations.** Most training programs will make accommodations for people with mental health problems. This step must be taken in advance, though, and may involve getting a note from a health care provider or counselor. Accommodations could include taking an exam in a separate room without others present or getting extra time. Think about what would be helpful and don't hesitate to speak up so that you get the help you need. Advocate for yourself!

Navigating Work

Before you navigate work, you need some work to navigate! Once you've tried to identify some of your interest areas and have a sense of your education, skills, and experience, it's time to start looking. This book is not intended as a guide to job hunting—once you are ready to start looking, I'd suggest finding local resources or a job coach. While it's great to look for and apply for jobs that you are keenly interested in, it's also good practice to submit lots of applications. Putting yourself out there gives you lots of opportunities to talk to people and, hopefully, have interviews. Below we'll focus on the aspects of work that are difficult for people with social anxiety.

PROBLEM: *I Have a Job Interview!*

While this is a good problem to have, job interviews create anxiety for almost everyone. Often, the more you want the job, the higher your anxiety will be. That's one of the reasons it's helpful to organize the informational interviews discussed above and put in a number of applications. The more interviews you do, the more confident you will feel.

SOLUTIONS

- **Prepare.** Once you've agreed to be interviewed, do some research about the workplace, employer, and interviewer. You may already have some of the information from when you put in your application, but it's good to be up to date and at least know the full name and position of your interviewer. Learn some facts about the goals and mission of the company, even if you're applying for an entry-level position. In that way, you will come across as well informed and interested.

- **Have questions ready.** Most interviewers will ask if you have any questions, so have a few in mind. It's good to have some general ones, such as "What's it like to work here?" or "Can you describe a typical day for this job?" or "What qualities are you looking for in an employee?" It's generally not a good idea to ask questions about salary near the beginning of the process.

- **Practice.** Have a friend, family member, or job coach help you by doing some role-play practices. Role plays can help you get used to interviews that start with straightforward questions and then proceed to more difficult questions. Put yourself in the role of interviewer a few times; this can sharpen your perspective and confidence. Ask the person you're practicing with for clear, specific feedback. "You did well" is positive, but hearing that you spoke too quickly, avoided eye contact, and appeared very uncomfortable can help you make improvements for the next role play and eventual interview.

• **Learn to be less humble.** Many people, particularly those with social anxiety, struggle to sing their own praises. In a job interview, it's very important to point out your skills, experiences, and positive attributes without denigrating them in any way. As children we are often taught not to "brag" so this may feel quite uncomfortable for you, but practice until it begins to feel more natural. There is no way an interviewer can know your strengths unless you point them out.

• **Turn it around.** A common interview question is "What would be one area that you need to work on?" It's often helpful to think of your response to this question in advance and put forward an attribute that can be spun in a positive direction ("I tend to work too hard" or "I have been told that I pull more than my weight"). Make sure you have also thought of a positive way to build on the issue you discuss.

• **Learn the eye contact trick.** People who are socially anxious often struggle with direct eye contact, but you can get around this by looking directly between the other person's eyes. This is easier than looking into the other person's eyes because it doesn't seem as intimate. The other person cannot tell the difference—it looks exactly like eye contact to them. Practice this strategy a few times and have someone else try it on you to see if you can see any difference. Be aware that this is clearly a safety behavior—a way to reduce your anxiety through avoidance. It can, however, come in very handy in some situations, including interviews.

• **Be gracious.** At the end of the interview, make sure you thank your interviewer and shake their hand. If appropriate, send an email note after the interview to let them know that you appreciated their time and questions. Some people with social anxiety are anxious about handshakes, so if this is the case with you, do some practicing.

PROBLEM: *I'm Starting a New Job*

You've worked hard on the application and interview process and have been offered and accepted a new job. You are very anxious as you will not only be learning all about the work and the company but meeting lots of new people. One of your thoughts is that it's important to make a good first impression, but you'd prefer to fade into the background and be quiet.

SOLUTIONS

- **Start with observation.** This may be relatively easy for a person with social anxiety. Observe others, get to know their names (write them down), and learn what their roles are. Notice the relationships among the people and who seems friendly and open.

- **Be friendly.** While it may be difficult, smile and say hello to everyone you meet and introduce yourself as the new person.

- **Keep your expectations of yourself reasonable.** Others will not expect you to remember everything and everyone or learn the ropes right away—it takes time as everything is new. Give yourself a break! Feel free to say "I don't know" when asked about company procedures, or "Who should I ask about that issue?"

- **Find a buddy.** There may be someone else who is relatively new or in a similar role to yours. If they seem friendly, ask them if it's okay to sit down with them and ask questions. It's always helpful if someone can guide you through your first few weeks, give you the "inside scoop," and perhaps become a new friend. They also could be someone you can sit with in the lunchroom or talk to at social events.

PROBLEM: *I Have a Performance Appraisal Coming Up*

After you've worked in a job for a few months, a performance appraisal is common and often part of the process of becoming a permanent employee. Appraisals do involve evaluation, both negative and positive. While they are routine, they can be anxiety provoking and have important consequences for your future.

SOLUTIONS

• **Keep a record.** When you start a new job or training program, keep notes about the work you do. These notes can include tasks that you take on and complete, comments received from others (customers, coworkers, supervisors), and times when you have helped others. If you have received positive comments, include quotes with dates attached to them.

• **Take responsibility.** If there have been issues with your work or schedule, keep track of this feedback as well and note any changes that you made to address these concerns. Do not shy away or try to avoid talking about problem areas. Have a plan for improvement or, if there are any ways that your supervisor could help, provide clear suggestions to them.

• **Avoid triangulation.** Do not, under any circumstances, mention or gossip about other employees during your performance appraisal (or during any other meeting for that matter). There may be times when this idea is tempting, such as "XX is also often late" or "I know that they received a raise"; talking about anyone else will, however, paint you in a bad light and put your supervisor in an awkward position. It is not your job to evaluate other people, so let your supervisor do their work.

• **Ask for specifics.** If your supervisor provides general feedback, either negative or positive, ask for examples or specific behaviors. For example, if they say that you're generally doing well in the job, ask what tasks you are doing well and how you could build on these tasks for the benefit of both yourself and the company. If you are given negative feedback, ask for examples and ask how you can address these issues. Let your supervisor know that you want to be a better employee. It's difficult to make improvements if you don't know exactly what to continue or to do differently.

PROBLEM: *I Want to Ask for a Raise*

Following a positive initial performance appraisal, you may be offered a permanent position, which may come with increased benefits or salary.

However, it may be up to you to ask for more money. Talking about money tends to be as difficult for many people as discussing sex and politics! But don't shy away from it—it's probably expected that you will at some point have a salary increase, but supervisors may hold off on offering it for as long as possible in order to save money for the company. On average, men tend to be more comfortable asking for a raise than women and on average are paid more.

SOLUTIONS

- **Do your homework.** It's helpful to know what the industry standard is for your job, as well as the salary of others who work in the same company or institution. It's very easy to undersell yourself when you're socially anxious.

- **Ensure that you ask for the going rate.** Once again, don't minimize or undervalue your services.

- **Don't apologize.** People who are socially anxious tend to apologize and be self-deprecating. Avoid giving your supervisor a rationale for declining to give you a raise by using statements like "I don't want to bother you" or "I know I haven't been here that long" or "I've heard that times are tight."

- **Be straightforward and direct.** Mention how you have added value to the workplace with examples provided from your performance appraisal. After noting your positive attributes, add some of the mutual benefits that you see moving forward and then ask for the increase in pay. Be ready with a specific request if asked. Also, be aware that if you have a positive review your employer may be willing to increase your pay or benefits. Consider that, depending on the circumstances, a raise could also include an increase in responsibilities or promotion in the role. Think about what you may be willing or unwilling to accept.

- **Follow up.** You may not be successful. Even if the answer is no, it's important that you have indicated to your supervisor what your request is. Make notes following the meeting and send your supervisor an email or note in which you thank them for their time. When you have your next performance appraisal, repeat your request.

PROBLEM: *Help! I'm Expected to Go to Networking Events*

Networking may turn out to be an important part of your job. These events can include conferences, business presentations, or sales calls but can also spill over into social situations such as company picnics, cocktail parties, or even sporting events. You may dread such events because they often involve meeting strangers and making small talk with people that you don't really know. Alcohol may be served, further complicating how to proceed. While it's tempting to avoid these events, your professional success may depend partially on being present and seen by others. The connections made could help advance your career.

SOLUTIONS

• **Find a colleague to connect with.** If you know someone else who is planning to attend the event, talk to them before you go and let them know you'll be there.

• **Set a time allotment.** Prior to going, decide on how much time you will spend at the event. Arrive shortly after it begins (but not early). Introduce yourself to a few people and ensure that others at your workplace see you there. Be sure to thank the host for the event. Don't feel obligated to stay too long, however. Leave when you planned and make a graceful exit. If you are feeling quite anxious about leaving, wait just a few minutes and then leave. Leaving when you are very anxious will reinforce your fears.

• **Remember that it's a work event.** Even though these activities take place outside of work and are social in nature, they are work events. Ensure that you keep appropriate boundaries in place for your behavior. For example, if your boss is drinking and starts flirting with you, be polite but firm in not flirting back. It's always a good idea to minimize alcohol consumption.

PROBLEM: *My Boss Is Taking Advantage of Me*

There are times when someone in a position of authority will put you in a difficult position. They may ask you to do inappropriate tasks, such as pick up their drycleaning on your lunch hour or gossip about a fellow employee. They may take one of your ideas and pass it off as their own. They may expect you to work after hours on one of their projects. Dealing with a difficult boss can be very challenging, as the potential consequence of being let go may be in the forefront of your mind.

> *Barry has worked as an instructor at a college for 10 years. He is hardworking and dedicated to his students. Last year he was involved in developing online courses that could be delivered internationally and potentially could boost the profile of the college. He was the key player on the committee although he tended to be unassertive in most meetings. He tended to work behind the scenes. He saw a brochure for a workshop about the courses that was to be presented by his boss at a conference. He checked the brochure carefully but saw only the name of his boss and the college. To add salt to the wound, the conference was at a beautiful resort in Hawaii! Barry was very upset. The material in the brochure was identical to what he had written and he was given no credit or opportunity for advancement for all of his hard work. His initial thought was that he would go challenge the boss directly, and then his next thought was that he would ignore it and quietly know that he had done good work.*

Neither of Barry's potential responses would be very effective! Dealing with potential conflict is difficult but a very critical skill to have in many situations.

SOLUTIONS

• **Have your documentation in order.** If your boss is taking advantage or even stealing your ideas, ensure that you have kept your work in case you need to provide proof to someone else. Have the facts in place prior to doing anything else.

• **Schedule an in-person meeting with your boss.** While it may seem unusual, try to have the meeting in a neutral space such as a meeting room rather than in their office. You will feel the power differential more strongly in their space than elsewhere.

• **Give them the benefit of the doubt.** Even if you are confident that they took advantage of the situation, it's not wise to challenge a superior directly with a statement such as "You stole my work!" A statement such as "I'm not sure if you're aware of the work that I did on this project" allows them an opportunity to ask questions or learn more about what led up to the development for which they are taking credit. Even if they were fully aware, it allows them to save face and propose a solution.

- **Be direct.** Review the principles of assertive communication and start with an *I* statement, such as (in Barry's case) "I see that you're presenting the new courses at the upcoming conference" and "I noticed that the names of the people on the committee were not included on the brochure, and I believe that it's important that we be given credit for our work."

- **State what you want to see happen.** Think about this step ahead of time and ask for it if at all possible. In Barry's case, this might entail asking his boss to prepare a slide listing the names of all the course developers and including them in all future communication.

- **Follow up.** Ensure that you send a written message after the meeting summarizing the discussion and what was agreed on. Document the meeting for yourself in case a similar situation happens in the future. Certainly, some bosses are unethical and take advantage, but some simply make mistakes and want to make amends.

- **Be kind to yourself.** Speaking up to someone in a position of authority is very difficult, and many people—not only those who are socially anxious—avoid doing it. Of course, avoidance is easier but not helpful in the long run. These kinds of patterns can persist and create a toxic situation. Another option is to have a confidential conversation with someone in Human Resources or a similar position. If you have a mentor outside of work who can advise you regarding potential solutions, that's also a good option.

PROBLEM: *I Want to Quit and Move On*

There are times when a job has outlived its usefulness and you want to do something else. Maybe a negative atmosphere has developed and you have been unable to influence it. Or you may be bored and would prefer new challenges. Many times, however, people remain in jobs out of fear of change and because they don't think they could do better. People with social anxiety and low self-esteem tend to undersell themselves, making it more difficult to take risks.

> Change can be liberating.

SOLUTIONS

- **Weigh your options.** Be realistic and make a chart of the pros and cons of remaining in your job. Are there options with your current employer that you would be interested in? At times an employer is keen to help employees advance their careers and help them learn new skills. But they won't do this unless they know you're interested in a change.

- **Network.** When you notice you are interested in a change, it is the time to call on your contacts. Reach out and invite some of them to have coffee and talk about the possibilities of new work. Ask for their discretion, particularly if your current workplace is not aware that you are looking for a change.

- **Remind yourself of your skills.** Just as in job interviews, it's important to sell yourself to yourself and not be modest. If you were a hiring manager, would you hire yourself? Why? Make a list of all the reasons that you'd make a great new employee.

- **Take a risk.** You are aware by now of the ease of keeping to the status quo and avoiding risk, but that keeps you stuck. Apply for some new positions and see what happens. You never know! Nothing can change without risk. Of course, it's easier to apply for jobs when you currently have the security of work, although this may not always be possible. Risk is a reminder that anxiety doesn't have to rule your life.

Most people have a number of different jobs during their working lives and learn from each and every one of them. Change builds confidence because with each new position you will be meeting new people, taking on new challenges, and building strengths.

Moving Forward

We have now reviewed numerous problems and solutions in the world of school and work. I hope you've already attempted some of the strategies—I am aware that many of the situations presented can be quite challenging for people with social anxiety. Standing up for yourself with a difficult boss, getting up to deliver a talk on your project, taking an exam, and having a job interview are things that you should be very proud of. Ensure that you give yourself lots of credit for any steps taken no matter how they work out. You don't have control over outcomes like influencing the boss or getting the job, but with gradual practice, persistence, and determination you can build confidence and be in charge of your own life.

10

keep it going

Congratulations! You've worked hard and come to the last chapter in the book. Hopefully you've learned a great deal and developed some new skills for living well alongside social anxiety. You have learned to challenge your thoughts and reduce avoidance as well as embrace who you are. No doubt you've tried some strategies and found some that work for you and perhaps some that do not. We are all unique and have different preferences, including those for change. Change is inevitable and constant, but it's important to take charge of it and keep it going in the direction you want.

At this point you may be surprised by your ability to do things that you couldn't do in the past. This happy outcome is likely the result of learning the strategies in this book and then practicing them. It's probably also the result of your starting to resist avoidance. Please keep that going too. When you come to the end of a difficult task or project, it's tempting to tell yourself that you deserve a break. But at the completion of a social anxiety group, I always warn clients against this temptation. Don't try to take a vacation from dealing with social anxiety. Every time you take a break, you'll probably have a setback and lose some gains.

It's very important to stick with this work over long periods of time. Confidence builds gradually with improved skills. And yet it's hard work! This chapter will focus on practical pointers to keep you moving forward.

Remember Your Goals and Values

If I had one piece of central advice, it would be to focus on your goals and what's most important to you. In Chapter 3 you identified your core values and set goals that were consistent with them. To keep progressing, it's crucial that you work toward goals that are aligned with your values. You'll likely lose interest if what you're trying to change is not that important or not in line with what you believe.

Here are some tips to keep up your progress with your goals:

- Review your goals regularly—they may shift over time.
- Review your values regularly—we often lose sight of what they are as we get caught up in day-to-day life.
- Keep the tips for goal setting in mind (this is a good time to review Chapter 3).
- Set new goals as you achieve the original ones.
- As you learn more about yourself, you will be able to fine-tune your goals.

Jorge had set goals of speaking at his cousin's wedding, giving reports at work, and volunteering to chair his monthly staff meeting. While he had been quite anxious, he felt very positive about meeting these goals. He was pleased that he had been able to say no to his cousin's request for money. He now had a much deeper understanding of his thoughts and avoidance patterns and realized how his problems affected his life beyond public speaking. He tended to hold back in conversations, was very agreeable, and seldom gave his opinion or initiated activities. Assumptions about how he was perceived by others dominated his thoughts, making spontaneity difficult. He decided that he wanted to continue to work on these problems and set goals for the future. While this included working on his original goals, he added goals of stating his opinion to his friends before he knew what theirs was, starting with noncontroversial topics, and progressing from there to other topics. He also decided to ask a group of friends to go on a camping trip for the long weekend that was coming up. He didn't know if they were interested in camping.

By setting the goal of asking his friends to join him on a camping trip, Jorge showed that he wanted to be fully spontaneous and in the moment, not distracted and distressed by anxious thoughts and a temptation to be influenced by them.

> **PRACTICE EXERCISE: Review your progress**
>
> Think back to your initial goals and answer the questions in the Social Anxiety Progress Review form on pages 207–208, recording your thoughts there or in a journal. (You can also download and print this form at *www.guilford.com/dobson3-forms*).

Keep Track of Your Progress

As you make progress, it's easy to minimize what you've done and dismiss it with comments such as "Most people can do that without difficulty" or "I should have been able to do that years ago; it's no big deal." It *is* a big deal, and you've worked hard. Keeping track of what you have done is rewarding and can be a visual reminder of progress. Earlier in this book I mentioned that it's a good idea to keep records of what you've done, including your challenges, thought records, and goals. Keep this habit up.

 • Chart your changes clearly so you can easily see what is happening. Keep your notes in a convenient place on your phone, laptop, or notebook and review them regularly for encouragement.

 • Consider ways to make the records visual, maybe with graphs. For example you could graph the number of situations that you now feel comfortable with, or your anxiety levels going down.

 • Keep a list of activities that you've tried and how easy/difficult they are (perhaps using a scale from 1 to 10, with 10 being the most difficult). Cross off the ones that are now quite easy—it's rewarding to cross items off a list!

 • Use reminders to help yourself keep track. Set reminders

SOCIAL ANXIETY PROGRESS REVIEW

What were your initial overall and specific goals?

Thoughts about your progress

Have you achieved what you hoped for?

How do you know?

Do you need to refocus or increase your efforts?

What are some of your future goals? Think about the short term (next few weeks), medium term (next few months), and longer term (next year).

What are some general tools that you have found helpful?

❑ Knowledge about social anxiety

❑ Understanding my own patterns and symptoms

❑ Realizing the consequences and costs of social anxiety

(continued)

❑ Knowing that avoidance helps in the short term but makes things much worse over time

❑ Breaking things down into components

❑ Creating distance to give me time to figure it out—slow it down

❑ Using my words—increasing my emotional vocabulary

❑ Realizing that my physical responses won't hurt me

❑ Seeing that we all wear different glasses and see the world through them

❑ Having a simple statement in mind, such as "Thoughts are just my opinion, not necessarily true"

❑ Learning to tolerate discomfort

❑ Doing what I fear, slowly and surely

❑ Practicing different types of social skills

❑ Being perfectly imperfect—embracing mistakes

❑ Customizing tools—making things my own

What are some tools you could use more often?

What are some tools you have not yet tried but might be helpful in the future?

regularly on your phone, either with visuals or sound. Put reminders in your physical environment. I like the use of "sticky dots" of your favorite color; no one else need know what they mean. For example, a red dot on your computer screen could be a "take a breath" reminder.

• Have a buddy if possible. Buddies can be a good source of positive credit as they will see things that you don't see and give you an external motivation to keep track and continue.

• Give yourself rewards for the work you've done. Rewards can be positive thoughts, comments to yourself or others, or physical rewards, such as an inexpensive gift (like a single flower) or watching a new series that you've been wanting to see.

Expect Ups and Downs

When I finish therapy with a client, I typically predict that they will have ups and downs to deal with, both positive and negative experiences. A life that is fully lived includes stressors, surprises, and setbacks. Remember that stressors can be good as well as bad. As you challenge yourself more and more, you will encounter opportunities that you might not expect, such as being offered a promotion that includes more responsibilities. Others may complain that you speak up too much when you previously were more complacent! Relationships often have complications and issues to deal with. You may be tempted to return to your old avoidance patterns, but resist, resist! Dealing with ups and downs is part of a life fully lived. The only life without stress is one full of avoidance.

> Lisa completed the program to become a personal trainer. Despite significant anxiety during her practicum training, she was able to tolerate being observed. She informed her instructor and had structured the tasks so that she proceeded gradually. She was very proud to obtain her certification. She was offered a part-time job in the local gym. On the first day of the job, she was assigned a very fit, high-profile client. While in her office observing the client and planning what she would do, she felt a panic attack coming on.

Her first thoughts were "Oh no, here we go again"; "I can't do this—I'm back at square one"; "I better quit now to save myself the embarrassment of showing him that I don't have a clue what I'm doing." Lisa immediately became discouraged.

As you can see, Lisa had a number of automatic thoughts that led her to want to avoid the situation and run away. In fact, it is very common and normal to reexperience symptoms from time to time. It would be unusual if these symptoms of anxiety never arose again. Think of how many years it took to develop your negative strategies (different types of avoidance, thinking patterns, complications) and how your environment sustained your anxiety. Think of how long it took for you to learn a complicated skill or a second language. Both took lots of time and energy. Anxiety is not going to go away in a flash and will try its best to gain a foothold. It's easy to go back to old habits.

If Lisa had declined the new job, she would not have had a panic attack and would likely still be stuck in her old job. But she wouldn't be doing something she loved, meeting new people, and feeling proud that she had pursued her dreams. Following are some strategies to try out when (not if!) something similar happens to you.

• **Don't be surprised.** If you expect setbacks, they will be less overwhelming and easier to manage. See setbacks as opportunities to hone your skills.

• **Watch your thoughts.** It's common to have thoughts such as "I'm back at square one," but that's an easy idea to challenge. It's impossible to be back at the starting point with all of the knowledge and experience you now have. You can never be there again. "Here we go again" is clearly a negative prediction and a misrepresentation of the facts, as the problems have not happened for quite a while. Use your thought record.

• **Create a plan.** Depending on what the setback is, it may be helpful to assess the situation from a distance and figure out a plan. Is it a major or minor setback? Should I pull back (rather than step out) and do something a bit easier? For example, Lisa could ask to be reassigned to a different client. Or she could ask for someone else to partner with her during the first session.

- **Give yourself credit.** The fact that you might experience some tension or anxiety likely means that you are pushing yourself or trying out new activities. In a sense, you are being brave and daring. Don't forget to recognize when you are pushing your own boundaries and be sure to give yourself credit for the effort.

Be Self-Compassionate

Accept yourself fully as you work hard toward meeting your goals. Acceptance and change are not incompatible. To accept yourself as a person doesn't mean that you embrace social anxiety. You can work on reducing problems while loving who you are as a person. You will make mistakes and be imperfect in your work on social anxiety as well as in other areas of your life. It's true for all of us. While I encourage you to keep trying and taking steps daily to live with your social anxiety, I guarantee that there will be days when this does not happen. You are human! Humans are not perfect (thank goodness!).

You are in a better position than anyone else to be compassionate and kind toward yourself. You know yourself best. Be kind and treat yourself the way you would treat a very good friend whom you love dearly. You may have had a lifelong habit of self-deprecation and, in fact, may have been quite mean in what you have said to yourself. If you've had a bad day, forgive yourself. It doesn't have to be a big deal— a day is just a day!

Here are a few tips to increase your self-compassion:

- Say the words that are going through your head out loud and see how they sound. Would you say them to a friend? If not, say something else.
- Practice being kind to yourself out loud with different words. Try out different phrases.

- Accept your humanity. Humans are imperfect. That is what makes us interesting.
- Use self-compassion meditation. A really good one is called "Loving Kindness"—you can easily find this brief meditation on YouTube or other media platforms.

Reach Out for Professional Help When Necessary

I hope that you've made progress by reading this book, learning all about social anxiety, and trying out the various strategies that have been presented. I'm thinking that you now have greater insight into your social anxiety and are living a more comfortable and confident life alongside it. During this journey you may have wondered about getting more help—it's possible that you've realized your problems could use a professional set of eyes, or that you've seen that you have developed some of the secondary issues that are hard to kick. It never hurts to get another opinion or reach out for therapy. Lots of people do, and we know it helps.

> *Ryan, the young man you met earlier in the book, kept living in his parents' basement. He continued to attend the monthly gaming meeting and met a few likeminded people. He had updated his résumé and sent it out to a few places but had not been invited to any interviews. He was feeling discouraged, and his mother commented that he was retreating into his shell again. He immediately became angry and lashed out at her. Shortly afterward he felt guilty. He knew from past experience that when he was feeling down he became irritable and had a short fuse. While he had tried some strategies to counteract his anxiety and learn social skills, he realized that he had a long way to go. He wondered about seeking professional help for his difficulties.*

There are times when trying something new leads you to realize that you don't have all of the tools you need. Maybe you'll decide you could use someone else to help you customize the tools for yourself. If you make this decision, the first step is most often to make an appointment with your primary health care provider or family doctor and talk to them about obtaining a diagnostic assessment. That would include a comprehensive interview to figure out what the problems are as well as their severity, other complications, risks, and strengths that you have. This type of assessment might involve completing a set of questionnaires to obtain more information. It probably would involve a referral for therapy (sometimes called *treatment*) and could include medication. We know from research evidence that medications and cognitive-behavioral therapy work for social anxiety.

As noted before, the most commonly recommended therapy for social anxiety is cognitive-behavioral therapy, or CBT. It is provided either individually (one on one) or in a group setting. Both formats work quite well and are relatively short term (usually eight to sixteen weekly sessions). If you live in a community with good resources, you could supplement individual CBT with a group CBT treatment or try them sequentially. This type of therapy is consistent with all the strategies in this book. It involves setting goals, trying out practical strategies, and doing homework assignments. The benefit of individual therapy is that it's more personalized and is likely to address any other problems that you may have, such as panic attacks or depression. The benefit of group therapy is that there is built-in social exposure every time you attend. Group therapy works best if all the other people also experience social anxiety and you learn and work together. There are significant benefits to being in a group, not the least of which is seeing that other people have similar struggles and that you are not alone. You learn from each other.

Other types of therapy are also available for social anxiety but have much less research support. Any therapy that strongly focuses on your past or that is primarily supportive in nature (for example, encouraging you to talk about your anxiety, but not encouraging change) is not likely to be effective and is not recommended for social anxiety. Be cautious about any therapy that discourages you from facing your fears and encourages you to avoid challenges. It will not help and could even make the situation worse.

Many people take medications for psychological problems. They are usually prescribed by your family physician or psychiatrist and are intended to be taken regularly. The most common medications for social anxiety are antidepressants. That may sound strange, but it was discovered that they work well for anxiety as well as depression. Lots of people take medications as well as participate in therapy—it's fine to do both at the same time. It is important to be aware that medications that simply reduce anxiety might incidentally also encourage you to avoid difficult or challenging situations. Think carefully about whether this is the approach you want to take. Anti-anxiety medication that is taken occasionally often works well for short-term stressful situations (such as a difficult airplane trip), but less well for longer-term anxiety problems such as social anxiety.

You may have had therapy in the past and, after reading this book, you may decide to give it another try. Situations change just as people do. It's useful to get help when you need it or if you simply feel like you'd like a "tune-up." We don't hesitate to take our vehicle in for a checkup or return to our family physician for an annual physical checkup. The same can be true for our mental health.

Look at the Big Picture

It's really important to look at the big picture. While everyday steps lead to progress, it's normal to make mistakes and have bad days. It's the overall change you make in your own life that counts. Don't let a down day lead to a series of down days. Sometimes it's easy to say "Well, I slipped up and didn't do anything yesterday, so I might as well not do anything today either." Watch out for this slippery slope! Progress is always up and down, and during times of transition, stress, illness, or other challenges, you may be less motivated and work less hard. That's okay.

Here are some tips to help you keep going over time:

• **Be persistent and consistent.** It's much more important to challenge yourself regularly with small steps than to try a big challenge occasionally. Before you know it, these small steps will seem easy and you will move on to the next step. While forgiving yourself for missing a day once in a while, take small opportunities that present themselves when in the past you might have avoided them. I call these *random acts of exposure*. Take advantage and be brave. Just like learning any new skill, regular practice builds a sense of accomplishment and increases your confidence.

- **Know your triggers.** Through the work that you have done so far, you probably know what the most difficult situations are for you, what your typical thought patterns are, what and how you avoid, and some of the more subtle avoidance behaviors you use. Before you read this book, you probably fooled yourself into thinking that these were good coping strategies, but now you know better! Your self-monitoring is important for understanding, and you probably won't be able to fool yourself anymore. This is a good thing. Awareness leads to change and helps you plan ahead.

- **Keep some structure in place.** Just as we have schedules for work, for school, and for other activities, consider keeping some structure for working on your social anxiety goals. You are more likely to continue if you know that every Sunday evening you will be planning your anxiety work along with your other weekly activities. Regular structure helps you build strong habits.

- **Keep motivated.** Progress makes a big difference in keeping you motivated. As you monitor and keep track of your progress, you will see positive changes, which is tremendously motivating and rewarding. Change is much more difficult at the beginning, but once you have reduced your avoidance, life becomes richer and more interesting.

I have had clients spontaneously report that as their lives became fuller and busier, they did something that previously had been difficult for them and they forgot to be anxious! They didn't worry in advance, and during the situation they were engrossed in it and didn't think about it until after it was over. I knew they were ready to complete therapy when it was difficult for them to fit in an appointment because there was too much going on in their lives. This is a terrific sign of progress, and it might happen to you.

Ending Reflections

I'd like to end this book with a reminder that I fully understand how it feels to experience social anxiety. I was a shy child and teenager and discovered I had a crippling fear of public speaking when I was a 17-year-old beginning university. I became skilled at avoidance strategies and was the quiet girl in the back of the class. Once I was in graduate school, however, I was forced to figure out how to overcome my fear. Luckily, I was in a clinical psychology program, so I knew the difficult steps I had to take. I learned how to give seminars and talk in classes where marks were given for participation. I signed up to teach undergraduate classes, which was the most difficult task of all. Teaching for six hours a week over the course of eight months did the trick. I discovered, however, after not teaching for a year or two, that my fear of public speaking had a habit of coming back. It took a long time for the fear to "go away"; however, I eventually started to really enjoy talking in public. There are still occasional circumstances when my anxiety may return, particularly when it's a personal situation such as at a wedding or funeral, but my anxiety in these cases is quite minimal. Even though my long journey may sound like a great deal of effort, it was all worth it; I value teaching and, as I've often said, if one can teach a class of 200 rowdy first-year students in college, it's easy to talk to just a few people!

I hope you'll continue to live your life fully alongside social anxiety. I think that over time you'll find social anxiety becoming smaller and smaller, less and less significant, and that life is becoming larger and more engaging, as it did for me and many other people. Just like some of my clients finishing therapy, I hope that you sometimes forget to be anxious because you are fully involved in what you are doing and living your best life. Knowledge reduces fear. Useful strategies increase confidence. Practice takes you out into the world of people, and social skills make you more comfortable in this world. With all of this, you can live well with social anxiety.

Index

about the author

Deborah Dobson, PhD, specialized in treatment of people with social anxiety disorder in her decades-long career as a clinical psychologist. Since retiring from clinical practice in 2023, she continues to provide training and consultation in cognitive-behavioral therapy, and is Adjunct Professor in the Department of Psychology at the University of Calgary. A recipient of the Governor General's Caring Canadian Award for her advocacy work in mental health, Dr. Dobson is a Fellow of the Association for Behavioral and Cognitive Therapies, the Canadian Association for Cognitive and Behavioural Therapies, and the Canadian Psychological Association.